GINSENG

GINSENG

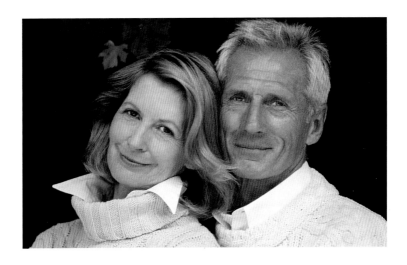

Stay Young & Vital

DR. ERNST D. PRINZENBERG

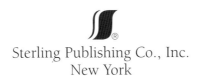

Sterling Publishing Co., Inc.
New York

Contents

**Library of Congress
Cataloging-in-Publication Data**

Prinzenberg, Ernst D.
  [Ginseng, Jung und vital ein
Leben lang. English]
  Ginseng : stay young & vital / Dr.
Ernst D. Prinzenberg.
    p. cm.
  Originally published in German
under the title: Ginseng : Jung und
vital ein Leben lang.
  Includes index.
  ISBN 0-8069-6571-1
  1. Ginseng—Therapeutic use.
I. Title.
RM666.G49P7513 1999
615'.32384—dc21   99–39011
                              CIP

10 9 8 7 6 5 4 3 2 1

Published by Sterling Publishing
  Company, Inc.
  387 Park Avenue South, New York,
  N.Y. 10016
Originally Published in Germany under
  the title Ginseng: Jung und vital ein
  Leben lang and © 1997 by Gräfe und
  Unzer Verlag GmbH, München
English Translation © 1999 by Sterling
  Publishing Co., Inc.
Distributed in Canada by Sterling
  Publishing
  C/o Canadian Manda Group,
  One Atlantic Avenue, Suite 105
  Toronto, Ontario
  Canada M6K 3E7
Distributed in Great Britain and
  Europe by Cassell PLC
  Wellington House, 125 Strand
  London WC2R 0BB, England
Distributed in Australia by Capricorn
  Link (Australia) Pty Ltd.
  P.O. Box 6651, Baulkham Hills
  Business Centre, NSW 2153,
  Australia

Printed in Hong Kong
Sterling ISBN 0-8069-6571-1

An Important Note

Ginseng is a natural remedy that has been used in Asia for many centuries. It has recently become popular in the Western world too, and is being researched by scientists. Ginseng strengthens the immune system and balances many bodily functions. It cannot, however, function as an all-round remedy for serious diseases, such as diabetes and cancer.

This guide describes various ways in which ginseng can be used and suggests appropriate doses. It is up to you to decide for yourself which ginseng product suits you best and what type of consumption you find most agreeable. The length of ginseng therapy varies from individual to individual as well. If you are undergoing medical treatment, inform your doctor or non-medical practitioner that you would like to use ginseng to support your treatment.

Preface

In ancient China, ginseng remedies were considered to be the finest means of treatment and to have long-lasting benefits. Completely without side effects, ginseng was used by people suffering from an illness or exhaustion to revitalize them and bring them inner harmony. The root of the ginseng plant was also thought to increase longevity and intensify zest for living.

Ginseng is the most commonly used medicinal plant in Asia. Only recently has this ancient, cultivated plant been rediscovered in the Western world as a remedy with numerous and diverse benefits. Ginseng has already been officially recognized as a general immunologic stimulant, as it supports the body and helps us cope better and more easily with harmful environmental influences. Ginseng has also shown its efficacy as an energy booster, quickly improving performance in business and in sports. In addition, it turns out to be a helpful adjunct in the treatment of diabetes and cardiovascular disorders. Ginseng has also proved to be equally suitable as a support in recovery from difficult surgery, in chemotherapy, and in preventive treatment against cancer.

Besides this abundance of benefits, ginseng can also have different effects depending on the situation. No matter what disorder or pain we may experience, one or another component will become effective, as if the remedy could think and feel on its own.

This guide will lead you through the history of ginseng—a history dating back thousands of years. It will also describe its contemporary methods of cultivation. The way ginseng grows and is processed has an important bearing on its quality and its active agent content. You will find many suggestions and tips on how to use ginseng and how to choose the products that are most appropriate for you. Whether you are young or old or somewhere in between, you can benefit from the power of ginseng—a power that fosters both harmony and strength.

Dr. Ernst D. Prinzenberg

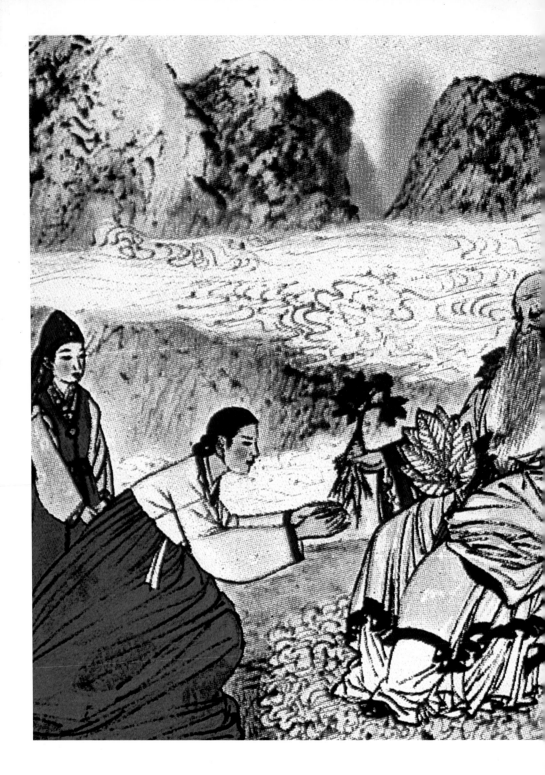

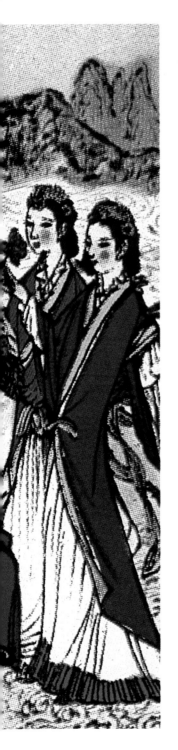

A Plant Reserved for Emperors

Chinese doctors have been using the root of the ginseng plant for nearly 5,000 years. Because of its healing power, it was much in demand and sometimes even more valuable than gold. In ancient China, ginseng was reserved for emperors; today, you yourself can take advantage of its numerous effects. The various kinds of ginseng differ greatly in quality. The curative power of ginseng depends on the way it is cultivated, the time it is given to grow and ripen, and the manner in which it is processed. Learn about the various kinds of ginseng, and find out what the real difference is between red and white ginseng.

The History of Ginseng

The ginseng root is called the "human root" because of its shape. Ginseng has been a part of Chinese and Japanese medicine for a long time. The plant is inconspicuous and consists of a stem, which is less than 3.28 feet (1 meter) high, and approximately six fingerlike leaves, which unfold in the shape of a hand. Ginseng grows mostly in the wooded mountains of China and Korea. Its long root is said to work wonders. Its shape resembles that of a human being, with parts that look like a head, arms, trunk, and legs or gown. The shape itself seems to indicate that the root is powerful enough to be effective in treating the entire human body. This is why ginseng has always captured the imagination of Asians. It comes as no surprise that numerous fairy tales, legends, and stories have been woven around this plant.

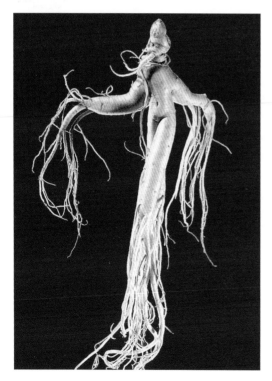

The Wondrous Effects of the Human Root

The Chinese named the root *jenshen* (ginseng), which means the "human root." The name consists of two words: *shen* (soul) and *jen* (the shape of man). The root is also known in China as *shen t'sao,* the soul herb. Koreans describe it as the Korean phoenix, *Poughwan.*

Ginseng Extends Life

According to legend, it was the ancient mythical emperor Shen Nung who discovered the wondrous root. He lived around 2700 B.C., and is considered to be the father of agriculture and herbal therapy. He is also credited as the author of the first pharma-copoeia, the *Pen-t'sao shen nung,* a book recounting the entire body of medical knowledge as it was known up to that time. Other Chinese medical books also testified to the fame and veneration that accompanied the potent root. These books said ginseng calms the mind, brings harmony to the soul, eliminates fears, and drives away evil spirits. It also makes the eyes shine, opens the heart, and clarifies thinking. If taken long enough, they claimed, it strengthens the body and extends life.

A remedy almost 5,000 years old

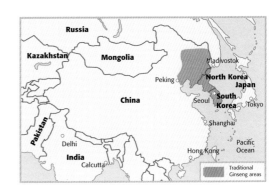

Place of Origin

The Chinese and the Koreans collected the ginseng root from the almost inaccessible woods of the mountain range that spreads from the Liaodang peninsula and the Jilin and Heilongjiang provinces in northeastern China through northern China all the way to the Pacific.

Even today, the best kinds of ginseng grow here.

What the Legend Says

A legendary remedy

Legend has it that the search for ginseng led ginseng pickers to almost impassable wooded mountains that were ruled by Sam, a mighty mountain spirit. Sam, or Samson, as he is known

The History of Ginseng

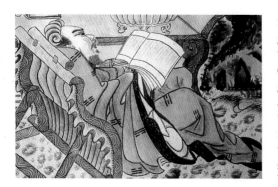

from the Bible, was a bearded god with flowing hair who, with his fearless tiger, guarded the entrance to where the ginseng was growing. According to the legend, only those with a pure heart could find the root; the others would have no luck in their search or would get devoured by wild animals in the woods. Mythical qualities

It hides deep in the woods.

Many stories are told about its fantastic strength. were also attributed to the plant itself: It glowed in the dark in order to show the way to the right hunter, but it could also hide itself in the ground when unwanted footsteps approached. Those who were successful in discovering the plant would shoot up an arrow, to mark the place where it was found.

Strength and Immortality

Ginseng was highly valued and much sought after. Possession and consumption of the root was associated in people's minds with ideas of strength and immortality. In Korea, ginseng was used as a means of payment close in value to gold and silver. From the fifth century on, wealthy Koreans made their tribute payments in ginseng. A century later, the same was done by the populations in the Kilin and Liaoning provinces, which today belong to China.

Along with the age and the composition of the root, its effectiveness also used to be categorized. The highest-quality roots were reserved for the emperor. Consumption of old roots from the best regions was at times even forbidden under penalty of death.

In 1711, the French Jesuit priest Pierre Jartoux gave a thorough report to his superiors about his encounter with ginseng during his journey through China: "Ginseng is too costly for the poor. It is an outstanding remedy for fatigue and excessive physical or mental exhaustion. It works as an expectorant, heals ailments of the lungs and the bronchial tubes, prevents vomiting, strengthens the stomach and stimulates appetite, lowers blood pressure, produces lymph in the blood, counteracts general indisposition, and prolongs life. If ginseng didn't possess all these qualities, it wouldn't be held in such high regard by the Chinese and the Tartars. Even healthy people take ginseng to strengthen their health. In my opinion, ginseng could become a wonderful medicine, if it gets into the hands of Europeans who know something about medicine and could conduct a study of the various ways in which it is effective."

Ginseng was held in the highest esteem.

Only today are Westerners in the position to conduct this kind of study and to make the royal remedy accessible to everyone.

Ginseng in Europe

The root was introduced to Europe in the middle of the ninth century by Arabs. The famous Arabic seafarer Ibn Cordoba supposedly brought the first ginseng roots to his homeland, Islamic Spain. Arabic scholars were thus aware of the healing powers of ginseng. But this knowledge was lost when King Ferdinand III conquered the province of Cordoba again. He ordered that all the captured ginseng roots be burned as tools of witchcraft. All of Eastern medical practice was condemned as the work of the devil.

Marco Polo brought ginseng from Asia to Europe.

A New Love Potion

Only in the epoch of the Enlightenment, at the beginning of the 18th century, did Europeans again take notice of ginseng. Just a scant knowledge of the effectiveness of the root had been preserved. People were, however, far less interested in the broad spectrum of its effectiveness than in its power as an aphrodisiac. The sailors could report about this, because ginseng had been used to increase sexual potency in the East for a long time.

Ginseng in the New World

A Jesuit priest who was familiar with Jartoux's reports (page 12) discovered a similar plant in Canada. Native Americans had used this plant for a long time for therapeutic purposes. The tribe of the Menomini called it *matcetasa*, "little Indian." The Ojibwa, who lived between Hudson Bay and Lake Superior, called it *shte-na-bi-o-dzhi-bik*, "man root."

Ginseng Intoxication

As a wild plant, ginseng has almost become extinct. The ginseng plant with its much sought-after root is pictured below.

News of the discovery of ginseng in Canada spread, triggering an enthusiastic search for the root. There was promise of great profits, as the demand for the royal root in Asia and increasingly in Europe was far greater than the meager supply on the market. And that is how the ginseng fever began. Within months, the stocks were plundered and the plant was almost completely eradicated, because nobody bothered to collect the seeds.

Soon ginseng became an important trade commodity in the United States as well. Large business firms transported ginseng to Europe and further to Asia. In 1862, as many as 620,000 kilos of ginseng were exported, at the price of up to 300 gold marks per kilo.

In 1749, according to some reports, not one grain harvester was to be found in the Montreal area; everybody had ginseng fever.

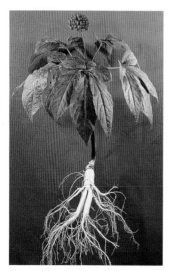

Ginseng Today

Over the past several decades, ginseng has once again aroused general interest. In the framework of holistic medicine, ginseng plays an important role (see page 28). The rising demand has led more than once to the falsification of its origin and age. Therefore, it's important for people in the Western market to know more about ginseng and the various ginseng products.

Wild Emperors and Red Kings

Today, wild ginseng plants are very rare in the impassable wooded mountains on the border between China and Korea. However, ginseng from plantations offers an economical alternative.

Modest and Hidden— the Ginseng Plant

Ginseng plants are also known by their botanical name: *Panaceae*. They belong to the family of Araliaceae and are related to ivy (*Hedera*). The part that is medicinally important is the root. It is long and narrow, and branches out in many smaller side rootlets. Its flesh is firm and white. Fine root fibers emanate from the side rootlets. The root can be up to 19 in. (50 cm) long.

Fresh ginseng smells like horseradish and licorice . It has a sharp, sweet, and, at the same time, slightly bitter taste.

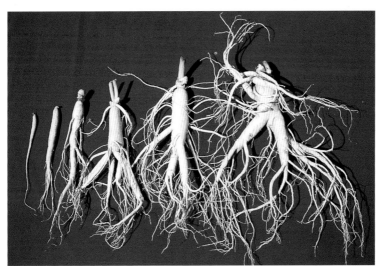

Ginseng roots are usually harvested when they are 7 to 11 in. (20 to 30 cm) long. Pictured, from left to right, are roots from one to six years old.

The Fleeing Plant

It takes between three and four years for ginseng to bloom for the first time. One flower umbel can carry as many as 80 pale green blossoms. Over the course of ripening, the fruit change their color from green to purple and then to deep red. Ginseng hunters thus speak of a "colorful rooster" or "firework fruit." In the fall, the blossoms wilt and the stem is shed. The following year, a new stem grows out of the bud on

The stages of growth the root neck. Every year a new bud comes forth, making the root neck a little longer. This way, the bud always appears on the

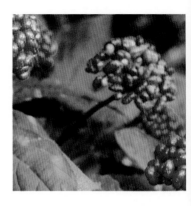

In its mature phase, it produces brightly colored fruit.

ground level, as the actual body of the root extends further into the ground. Because of this, the root is described as "hiding from people." As it grows, the root acquires constrictions, which look like annual rings and help determine its age.

The Homeland of Ginseng

Ginseng's original homeland is the great forest area in the temperate climatic zone between the 38th and the 48th parallels—that is, between Seoul in South Korea and Jiamusi in northeastern China (see also page 11). Ginseng grows on nutrient-rich, well- aerated, and water-storing soil in areas that are between 656 and 3,608 feet (200 and 1,100 meters) high. It prefers the shade and a high level of humidity in the air. Ideal summer temperatures are between 68 and 77 degrees F (20 and 25 degrees C); ideal winter temperatures are from 39 to 57 degrees F (1 to 14 degrees C).

Korea and Northern China

Mountain Ginseng, the Old Sage

Of the different types of ginseng, wild ginseng is the highest in terms of quality and is the rarest and most esteemed. Its demanding character limits its biotope to a narrow strip of land around the 40th parallel. There, it grows slowly, on its own, in the im-passable mountains of China and Korea. As with good wine, it takes a long time for ginseng to ripen and for its constituents to balance each other out in a way that produces the best possible effects. There have been reports of roots 200 years old. The sign of its aging process is the small wrinkles on the root skin. Unfortunately, its healing powers and the unceasing demand for it have almost completely wiped it out. There are still no laws that protect the remaining wild ginseng plants from being eradicated.

Long ripening is important.

Imperial Ginseng, a Close Second

There have been many attempts to build up ginseng's natural habitat in the wooded mountains. Ginseng hunters would take the seeds with them and plant them in the places where ginseng had grown or could grow. The roots of the plants that grew from these seeds were called "imperial ginseng," because roots of this quality belonged in former times to the emperor of China. Imperial ginseng bears a resemblance in shape to that of wild ginseng, but its quality is not quite the same. Imperial ginseng is, nonetheless, one of the most valued ginseng products.

Especially valuable, imperial ginseng used to be the root of emperors.

Cultivated Ginseng

The demand for ginseng has always been great. Under cultivated conditions, ginseng grows faster but its period of growth is limited. The cultivation is lengthy and demanding on the part of the planter. Unlike wild ginseng roots, the roots of cultivated ginseng are stocky and meaty and their skin is youthfully smooth.

All Ginseng Types Are Not Created Equal

Ginseng is cultivated all over the world today. Ginseng comes from Korea, China, Japan, Thailand, Russia, and Canada. This could lead one to the false impression that ginseng from all these countries is the same but just with a different place of origin. However, different kinds of ginseng are cultivated in different areas. They all belong to the family of Araliaceae, but they differ in their content of active agents, in their distribution pattern of individual active agents, and therefore in their overall effectiveness. Unfortunately, the considerable variations among different kinds of ginseng are generally not well known, and this is why various products used to be sold under the same name even though their effects were quite different. Consequently, ginseng lost its reputation as the royal remedy. Only two kinds of ginseng are medicinally considered genuine: the Chinese-Korean *Panax ginseng C. A. Meyer* and the Canadian *Panax quinquefolius*.

There are different kinds of ginseng.

Panax Ginseng C. A. Meyer

Panax ginseng C. A. Meyer, named after the German-Russian botanist Carl Anton Meyer, who was the second Westerner to describe in detail this kind of ginseng, is considered to be genuine and can be used for medical purposes. It is the most valuable, the best known, and the most heavily researched type of ginseng.

The king of herbal remedies

The growth requirements of *Panax ginseng C. A. Meyer* limit the geographical area in which it can grow.

Because of the diversity of its active agents and the richness of its effects, *Panax ginseng C. A. Meyer* is also described as the king or the emperor of herbal remedies. As a wild plant, it is hard to find and almost extinct. To protect its wild habitat, people tried very early to cultivate this type of ginseng. The ideal soil quality and a suitable climate were found in northeastern China (Manchuria) and in Korea, which were the traditional Asian ginseng-growing areas and where the roots had always shown their best qualities (see page 11). For the sake of simplicity, we will use the term "ginseng" when referring to *Panax ginseng C. A. Meyer.*

Imperial ginseng is the best emulator of the "wild emperor."

Cultivated Kings—Imperial Ginseng

In certain places, for instance on the Chinese-Korean border, ginseng plants are still cultivated as if they were growing wild (see page 17). The roots of this plant are sold at very high prices as "imperial ginseng." The roots of plants cultivated on plantations and six years old or older come close in value. They are offered as "red ginseng" (see page 25), which is not a different kind of ginseng but rather a special, high-quality root of *Panax ginseng C. A. Meyer.*

Panax Ginseng Quinquefolius

The closest relative of the real Chinese-Korean ginseng is *Panax ginseng quinquefolius.* Native Americans already used it for medicinal purposes. It possesses a great number of certain constituents, lacks some altogether, and differs from the Asian ginseng in its composition.

Plantation growth in southern Canada and northeastern United States

Ginseng's Other Relatives

● *Panax pseudoginseng*
This is a distant relative that is used for medical purposes in China, Vietnam, and the Himalayan region. Wild specimens of this kind, san-tchi ginseng, have a long growing period and are very valuable. They can still be found, although rarely, in India, Nepal, and Myanmar.

● *Panax japonicus*
A Japanese type of ginseng, it is a subspecies of *Panax pseudoginseng,* and not only can be found in Japan but also in China, Vietnam, and Thailand. Its healing powers, however, do not measure up to the standards of the real ginseng.

● *Eleutherococcus senticosus*
This kind of ginseng is also known as "Siberian ginseng." Externally, it is quite different from the real ginseng. It is found in Russia, China, Korea, and Japan. Instead of ginsenosides (page 36), it contains eleutheorsides. In the seventies, it was used in Germany as a substitute for the rare and thus expensive real ginseng and was known as the "taiga root."

None of these kinds could gain the worldwide stature of the real ginseng.

Cultivated Ginseng from Plantations

Since ginseng began to be cultivated, its biotope has spread widely. The cultivation of ginseng is particularly intensive in northern China and Korea, where the conditions are especially favorable.

Ginseng Loves Shade and Moisture

Ginseng prefers a moderate or continental climate and the natural vegetation of deciduous woods in mountainous areas. Particularly valuable plants (for instance, red ginseng, see page 25) grow on the gently rising northern and northeastern hillsides, between 1,312 and 3,280 feet (400 and 1,000 meters)

Ginseng needs constant moisture.

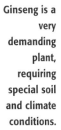

Ginseng is a very demanding plant, requiring special soil and climate conditions.

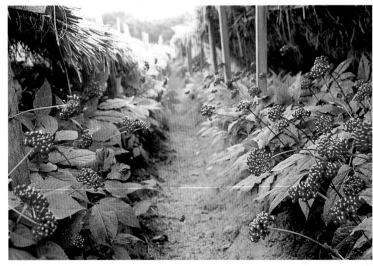

high, from which precipitation water can be drained for irrigation. Ginseng needs to be watered regularly. It should not, however, stay wet. If it does, its roots will rot in the soil.

Lower-quality types of ginseng, such as white ginseng, are grown in areas that get a great deal of sun exposure and from which water cannot be easily drained. Because ginseng prefers

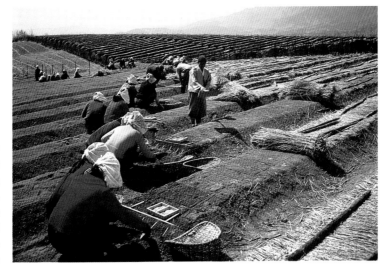

Plots for high-quality ginseng are costly, because they need to be cultivated by hand.

the shade, and most plantations do not have foliage as a natural cover, special pergolas that cast off 80 to 90 percent of the direct sunlight need to be constructed.

It Takes a While to Do Something Well

The cultivation of ginseng requires a great deal of time and work. Ginseng is cultivated from the seeds of four-year-old plants. Germinated seeds are scattered over the shaded seedling plots and covered with sand. In order to sprout, the seeds need to be watered regularly and kept free from weeds and pests.

The seeds need from one and a half to two years to sprout. Then a short stem with one leaf develops. The little plant receives a supply of nutrients from a mixture of soil and natural fertilizers. At the end of the year, the withered stem and leaf are

It is said that "ginseng likes to hear the steps of the gardener every day."

Cultivated Ginseng from Plantations

removed by hand and the plot is covered by mulch in order to withstand the rigors of winter.

Attentive Care for the Soil and Plants

After three years, the seedlings are carefully dug up and re-planted into plots for growing. For two years before that, the soil in the plots is carefully prepared to take up the tender and demanding little plants. It is ploughed up to 15 times, and each time a certain amount of wild-growing grass is added.

The young plants are then replanted two more times into the shaded, straw-covered plots. The crop has to be protected from sunlight and from pests. It needs to be watered regularly and fertilized using a cleverly devised system.

After four to six years, and usually around the end of September, the root is dug up from the soil with utmost care so as not to damage the delicate root fibers. Afterward, it is carefully washed by hand and the soil is removed with fine brushes. The roots are dried on large sundecks. High-quality roots are usually preserved immediately, because ginseng roots rot easily. (See red ginseng, page 25.)

Ginseng roots are dried in the sun.

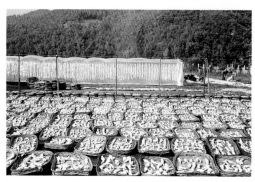

Planters have to invest a great deal of time and effort over the four to six years between planting and harvest. Ginseng cultivation is still often done exclusively by hand. The cultivation soil requires about 10 years to regenerate completely. This means that high-quality ginseng can only be harvested about every 16 years.

High-quality roots are only harvested every 14 to 16 years.

The Quality Lies in the Root Fiber

For trading purposes, each root is inspected separately and categorized according to its size, appearance, and subsequent quality. The highest content of active agents is found in the largest and strongest roots with the most pronounced and best preserved delicate root fibers. (See also page 37.)

Ginseng as an Economic Factor

Making high profits with ginseng

As the most heavily used herbal remedy in Asian medicine, ginseng is a significant trade product. Korea alone exports more than 70 million dollars' worth of ginseng per year.

Consequences of a Monoculture

Ginseng, like other agricultural products, is cultivated in many areas in large monocultures. There, the priority is not the quality of the ginseng but rather its greatest possible economic usefulness.

In order to increase the yield, the traditional field regeneration period, which was formerly 10 to 12 years, has been shortened to only two years. For instance, this is the case in cultivation areas in Russia and some parts of Korea. The root's frequent rotting is perhaps a way nature reacts to the unnatural conditions of planting a single crop. In monocultures, pests can often be combated only with chemical substances (pesticides).

Pests are fought with pesticides.

Importance of the Origin

Some quality-conscious producers, however, use a method of producing dried medications and extracts that makes it possible to preserve the active agents without pesticide residues. For this reason, when buying ginseng products, you should inquire not only about the origin of the product but also about its processing techniques (see "The Range of Ginseng Products," page 40, and "How to Buy Ginseng," page 51).

In some countries, ginseng is not pharmaceutically controlled.

In addition, it is not advisable to buy cheap remedies without knowing where they come from, how they were processed, and which ingredients they contain. In the United States, Great Britain, and Australia, for instance, ginseng is not categorized as a medical plant but rather as a health food. Ginseng products in these countries are not subject to the laws of pharmaceutical control. Therefore, ginseng products that are sold there may more frequently contain higher residues or harmful additives. Some of the products that were examined contained no active agents whatsoever (see "Ginsenosides," page 36).

Red Ginseng and White Ginseng

Different products

Red and white ginseng are not different types of the same plant, as is often assumed. They are rather two different products of the same plant, which are preserved in different ways and exhibit different quality features.

Red and white ginseng both come from *Panax ginseng C. A. Meyer* (page 18), the highest quality of which originates in northern China and Korea. Roots of very high quality are se-lected to prepare the much sought-after and especially valuable red ginseng.

Young and White

Four-year-old roots from the plains

More often than not, the plants from the plains are harvested when they are four years old and treated as white ginseng. Because fresh ginseng can quickly deteriorate, it is sun-dried and rapidly processed. The roots appear yellowish-white. As a dried root or powder, this product is labeled on the market as "white ginseng" or simply as "ginseng."

It becomes
red through
a special
method of
preserva-
tion.

Like a Red Crystal

Red ginseng is produced from the high-quality, six-year-old plants from the highlands. The name "red ginseng" is no feature of the plant itself but rather a reference to a very old and efficient technique that makes ginseng keep well.

As a rule, red ginseng has a highly concentrated active agent content (see page 36). The harvested roots are kept fresh naturally with steam. In this way, a chemical process known as the Maillard reaction is activated. This reaction is responsible for making the roots red. They also become hard and resistant. With this form of preservation, the active agents are kept intact. Following this, the roots are dried. They acquire a red-orange color and become crystalline or have a hornlike transparency.

Red ginseng is usually processed further as an extract or an extract powder. The dried and ground root is also available in powdered form either loose or in capsules (see drug products, pages 40 and 53).

White Ginseng	*Red Ginseng*
● Derived from plants that are three to four years old	● Derived from six-year-old plants
● Cultivated mainly in the plains	● Cultivated in the higher, high-quality regions
	● Distance stipulated between the plants, which are planted next to each other, in order to achieve the maximum content of active agents
● Preserved by bleaching and drying	● Preserved by steaming and drying
	● Development of further active components, such as maltol
● Yellowish-white coloring	● Orange-red coloring

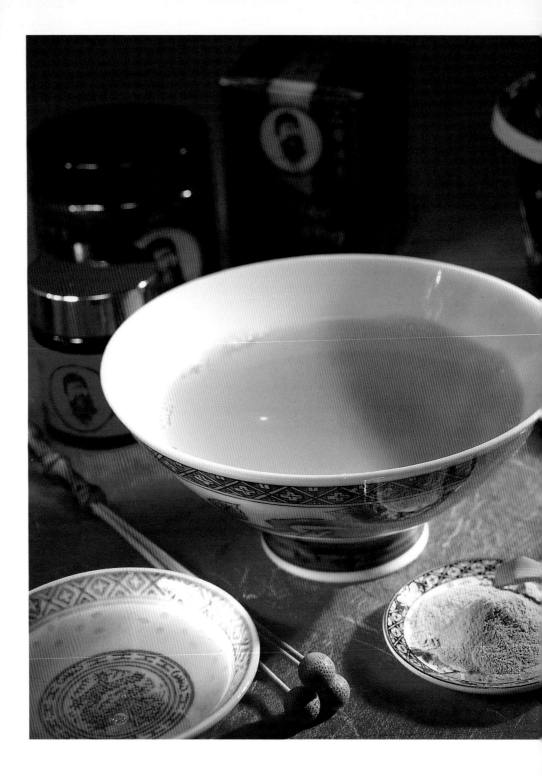

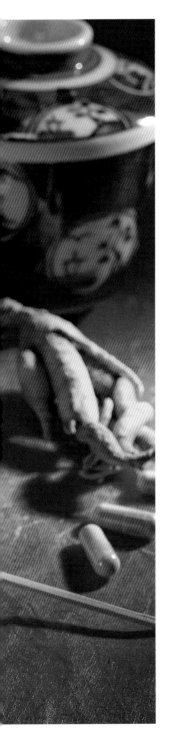

Ginseng— Effects and Dosage

Health is, according to Chinese doctors, the equilibrium of body and soul. Ginseng is a remedy that in many ways helps in creating this equilibrium and in eliminating disturbances in bodily functions. In doing so, it can adjust its effects to the needs of the individual. This almost unique harmonizing effect is based on the ingenious interplay of ginsenosides, the special active agents of the ginseng root.

There are numerous ginseng products on the market, of differing quality. However, a few simple tips can help you discover the best products for yourself and the best ways of taking them.

In Harmony with Body and Soul

Seeing humans as complete beings again

For a long time, Western medicine, as a standard academic subject oriented toward the natural sciences, had a narrow focus: researching separate clinical issues and curing the symptoms of diseases. Furthermore, in many places, it has turned into an expensive kind of "equipment medicine," the cost of which society is barely able to tolerate any longer. Human beings, as both physical and psychological entities, have receded into the background. Measures to maintain health and prevent diseases have not received proper attention. However, naturopathy has proven to be a valuable asset in these areas. Standard Western medicine and naturopathy can also complement each other in the treatment of diseases. Along with a growing interest in holistic medicine over the last couple of decades, there has also therefore been a growing interest in traditional Chinese medicine.

Chinese Medicine

Chinese medicine, as opposed to Western medicine, does not focus primarily on the treatment of a disease but rather on that of the whole person. The unity of body, psyche, and soul thus emerges to the foreground. In order to eliminate the symptoms of a disease, an attempt is made to restore the balance of the afflicted organism as a whole. In addition, the self-curing mechanisms of the individual need to be set in motion. Another important objective is disease prevention. In earlier times, the most highly esteemed doctors were those whose patients did not get sick in the first place. Traditional Chinese doctors primarily use herbal remedies, which they administer in many combinations.

Health equals balance.

Various active agents complement one another and often produce a cumulative effect, which cannot be explained through scientific methods of investigation. Recently, Chinese medicine, or at least some of its treatment methods, have been acknowledged by many Western-trained doctors, especially as an adjunct to standard medical practices or as a means of preventing diseases.

An Ancient Tradition

Chinese herbal medicine has a long history. It goes all the way back to the early Han era, or the second century B.C. The effects and side effects of various remedies have been carefully observed over many generations. There were 365 remedies listed in the medical directory of those days, the *Pen-t'sao shen nung* (page 11), with each of them corresponding to one day of the year. The remedies were divided into three groups, which differed in the scope of their effects and side effects.

Ginseng as a Master Medicine

The first 120 remedies supposedly have no side effects. They maintain and strengthen the body without weakening or harming it. They are called royal remedies, because kings are, or at least should be, concerned about the overall well-being of their people. Ginseng is the master of this group, as it can restore harmony in a special way, works gently but reliably, and is supposed to have no side effects.

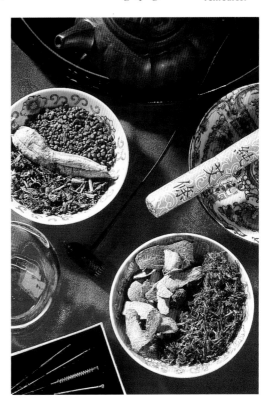

Ginseng occupies an important position in the diverse world of Chinese herbal remedies.

The ministers: only for certain diseases

● The middle group also contains 120 remedies. These can be poisonous but only to a minor extent. They are called ministers, because they, too, preserve the community, although this does not always happen for solely selfless reasons. They prove to be effective but sometimes appear "vain and stubborn." Their effectiveness is limited to certain disease forms, their usage requires supervision, and they are only advised for a limited period of time.

● The remaining remedies are known as assistants. They perform concrete jobs but always require guidance from a learned master. Their effectiveness is limited in time, and they are only used for a specific situation. Although these remedies are good for focused applications, they are usually tough and cannot balance the whole organism. They are used for quick improvement of certain acute symptoms, like fever or shivers. Because they are usually quite poisonous, they should be used only in emergencies.

The assistants: only for emergencies

How to Find the Right Remedy

● Royal remedies support the internal harmony of the body,
● ministers support cyclic transformations in diseases, and
● assistants cause simple developments, such as the reduction of fever.

Unity through Difference—Yin and Yang

Yin and Yang are not opposing forces—they belong together. We carry both aspects in us.

Light and shadow or ebb and flow only appear to be opposites. They in fact belong together and require each other, like day and night, wakefulness and sleep, youth and old age, and hot and cold. Without pain, there would be no joy, without death no life. These different manifestations of the same principle dominate our entire existence. Without them, our lives would be unimaginable. The Chinese call these two sides yin and yang. Yin and yang are thought of as the two sides of a coin, and they represent two aspects that are only imaginable together. Originally, yang was the sunny side of a mountain, or the south, whereas yin was the shadowy side, or the north. But now each contains many more meanings and classifications.

● Yin describes the reclining, existing, dark, feminine aspect, whereas

● yang describes its complementary dynamic, the developing, bright, masculine aspect.

Only together do they make up a whole.

But yin and yang are also related to each other: Yin can shelter yang, and vice versa.

Everything Changes

The appearances of yin and yang change. Through non-change, transformation, and metamorphosis, all things and beings manifest. The cycle of change from the summer and the rule of light to the lack of light in the winter is contained within the eternal change of yin and yang, as are the attraction between masculine and feminine natures and the course of coming into existence, maturing, and aging. Within the changes of yin and yang, the cosmos completes itself.

Yin and yang constantly change.

Yin and yang work on a large cosmic scale in the same way as they work together within the small world of the human organism. According to traditional Chinese thought, bodily processes go through the same changes and transformations of yin and yang, If yin and yang are in equilibrium, this leads to overall well-being. If they are out of balance, problems and diseases occur.

● **Non-change** implies a standstill, disturbances, and complaints, which limit our ability to handle tasks in daily living (see page 61).

● **Transformations** are phases of great burdens, such as when we are ill, during which the body has to fight for its equilibrium (see page 73).

● **Metamorphosis** describes the processes of maturing that we go through over the course of our lives; examples are menopause and aging (see page 89).

In Harmony with Body and Soul

Ginseng, a Source of Harmony

Holistic thought, which also includes Chinese medicine, has a much clearer idea of health than we have in our world of comprehension, where we often define health only as the absence of symptoms. Being healthy primarily means living in unison with a natural and divine rhythm, and thus being aware of the "right time" and the "right place." Being in sync this way, the individual experiences internal and external harmony. This is the most important goal.

Internal and external harmony fosters health and strength.

A Refined Interplay of Active Agents

Ginseng is special in that it can influence the human body in so many ways that it can adjust to a certain situation in the best

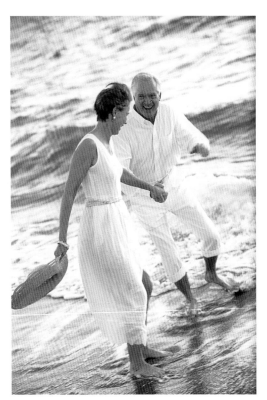

possible manner, thereby restoring the balance of the body. Through the interaction of its active agents, ginseng can bring about harmony in all bodily organs. Thus, it helps to keep the whole human being healthy and properly "centered." It is invigorating for the body and the psyche, and it stimulates the brain. Such balancing, holistic effects have only been observed in a few and often related kinds of plants, although usually in a less pronounced manner. Ginseng is not known as the king of remedies without reason. In Chinese medicine, ginseng is therefore a component of many different remedies.

How Ginseng Works

Ginseng strengthens the whole organism.

Ginseng doesn't work in only one direction. It adjusts itself to the individual human being and his or her current needs:

● People who are stressed or under pressure are helped to mobilize their reserves and use them as effectively as possible. Ginseng improves their performance and relaxes them at the same time.

● People who are exhausted and without motivation are helped to regenerate more quickly and develop new energies.

Protection and Regulation

Ginseng can help to make blood pressure either higher and lower, depending on the situation that it is used for and whether the patient's blood pressure is too high or too low. The well-known ginseng researcher Dr. Israel Brekhman has coined the term "adaptogenic" (from the Latin *adaptare*) to describe this kind of effectiveness that is adaptable to the patient's needs. This special effect of some plants can be explained biologically by the fact that they contain a mixture of active agents that can become more or less active depending on the patient's constitution.

Ginseng can have a normalizing effect on altered organic functions.

Adaptogens—Remedies That Adapt to Needs

Plants that work adaptogenically:

● improve the body's immune system and thus help us adjust to internal and external pressures,

● influence the altered conditions of the body positively, regulating and normalizing them, and

● are without harmful side effects, so they can be used without a second's thought.

How Ginseng Works

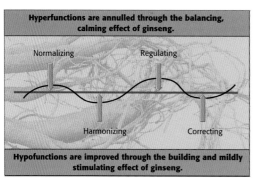

Hyperfunctions are annulled through the balancing, calming effect of ginseng.

Normalizing   Regulating

Harmonizing   Correcting

Hypofunctions are improved through the building and mildly stimulating effect of ginseng.

If the sugar level in the blood gets too high or too low, ginseng corrects this value to a relative optimum, by increasing or decreasing the sugar level. Should there be pressure from the outside that causes a sudden drop in the sugar level— for example, when insulin is administered—the body can react to it better and more quickly. It is assumed that gin-

The active agents of the ginseng root harmonize the activities of the body.

seng remedies change the functioning of the metabolism in such a way that more hormones of the reducing metabolism are produced in advance. The organism can then react better should the need arise. In a person with balanced sugar levels in the blood, ginseng does not have an immediate effect.

Therapeutic effect as required— just what the individual needs

Avoiding Internal and External Attacks

The same holds true for the immune system. When the human body has been prepared by ginseng, it is able to provide the necessary defense cells more quickly and effectively and can defend itself against internal and external pressures. Internal, metabolism-related fluctuations are absorbed or eliminated. This is how the detoxifying work of the liver and the balancing of the fat content in the blood are supported. Environmental pollution by harmful chemicals, toxic substances, and even radioactivity can be tolerated much more easily by the organism. Not only does ginseng absorb important substances more quickly, but it also rapidly excretes the harmful ones.

Ginseng strengthens the powers of resistance.

Effective Help in Everyday Life

Ginseng is not a magic substance that can heal all diseases. Medical measures are necessary and important when dealing with serious illnesses. Frequently, however, we can support these treatments with ginseng. But it is when we are trying to cope with the diverse and small knocks of everyday life that ginseng is especially effective.

Every Root—an Abundance of Active Agents

In every root, various substances can be identified, and every single one of them is linked to particular effects. For example, one constituent lowers blood pressure and another causes the opposite effect.

Strength from the soil

What represents a mysterious jigsaw puzzle for the Western pharmacologist remains a gift of nature for the Eastern practitioner—a gift whose healing and strengthening influence has been shown and proven through many years of experience. The individual active substance does not determine the healing power of ginseng; it is rather the sensitive interplay of all the substances taken together.

A wealth of healing power and life energy is contained in these roots.

A Remedy with Royal Demands

Because ginseng is effective in so many different ways, it is easy to understand why the soil, climate, region, and care during cultivation play such important roles. Unlike fast-growing arable crops, more than one factor is significant. Many different active agents have to be developed and to remain balanced in relation to one another at the same time. The best and most balanced spectrum of effectiveness can only develop if the plant grows under optimal conditions (see page 20). This royal plant is as demanding and fragile as a princess.

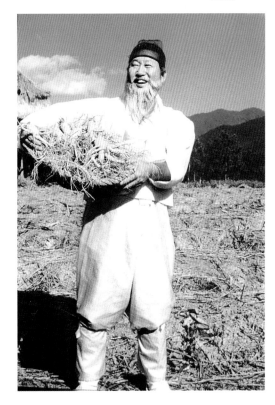

Ginseng's Active Agents

Diverse ingredients

The diverse and seemingly contradicting effects of the ginseng root naturally aroused the curiosity of chemists. In numerous experiments and analyses, they have tried to determine the individual constituents.

General Constituents

● Fats and ethereal oils; proteins and their components; vitamins, such as B-12 and the A vitamins; choline; mineral salts, such as sodium and magnesium; and trace elements, such as boron, manganese, and iron, have been discovered.

The discovery of specific ginseng ingredients

● Ginseng also contains vanadium, selenium, fluorine, and germanium. The effects of selenium and germanium have recently been discussed as possible "factors of cancer protection."

● Ginseng also contains 5 percent glucose, which gives it a sweetish taste.

Ginsenosides have been researched worldwide.

However, none of these active agents are counted among the main active agents. They may have a supporting role in ginseng's effectiveness, but they cannot explain its special healing power. During the sixties, a group of scientists in Moscow discovered a group of chemically related substances in ginseng, called ginsenosides.

Ginsenosides

Ginsenosides belong to the group of saponins. If ginseng powder is shaken with water, a layer of froth develops, like when soap is beaten in water. The froth is easy proof of the presence of saponins (in Latin, *sapo* means soap). Saponins are widespread in the plant kingdom. They are among the most important defense substances in plants against infections.

Ginsenosides

Main Ginsenosides
Rb1, Rb2, Rc, Rd (group of panaxdioles)
Rg1 and Re (group of panaxtrioles)

Other Ginsenosides
Rb3, Ra1, Ra2, Ra3, Rg3, Rh2, Rs1, Rs2 (panaxdioles)
Rf, Rg2, and Rh1 (panaxtrioles)
Ro (group of oleanolic acids)

The saponins that are present in ginseng, the ginsenosides, consist of sugar parts and a nucleus that is vaguely reminiscent of steroid hormones, such as estrogens. The ginsenosides are considered to be the primary active component of the ginseng root. To this day, 28 different ginsenosides have been isolated and analyzed for their chemical structure. There are primarily two large groups with different sugar parts: the panaxdioles and the panaxtrioles. In addition, there is also a representative of oleanolic acid.

The main active agents of ginseng

How Ginsenosides Are Distributed

Ginsenosides are formed in the flowers, leaves, and root skin of the ginseng plant. From there, they move to the root, where they are stored. The climate, soil, and quality of the seeds determine how many ginsenosides will develop.

Ginsenosides are not distributed equally throughout the root. The main root contains a rather small percentage of ginsenosides, whereas the ginsenoside content of the side roots is approximately three times higher, and that of the root fibers as much as 10 times higher. Therefore, the roots have to be removed and processed very carefully so as not to injure the valuable root fibers.

The ginsenosides are also distributed unevenly in other parts of the plant. In American ginseng, for example, the representatives of the Rf-group are almost exclusively contained in the leaves, the Reconnection is mostly in the flowers, and a large amount of Rg1 can be found in the root.

The ginsenosides are distributed in a very distinctive manner in the root. Here is a cross-section of red ginseng.

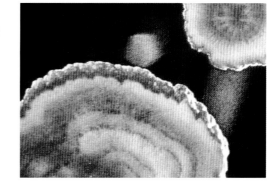

Knowing the Differences in Quality

It is impor-
tant to
understand
how gin-
senosides
are distrib-
uted and
how they
work
together.

The amount of ginsenosides in the plant, as well as the pattern in which the individual ginsenosides are distributed, and the way they complement each other, depend mainly on the kind of ginseng. American ginseng differs from Korean ginseng in that it has a larger amount of certain ginsenosides but not the whole spectrum of ginsenosides. The different ginsenoside profiles are responsible for the quality and the healing power of the root. Not only the amount of ginsenosides, but also the ratio among them, is important as a determinant of its healing power.

How Ginsenosides Work

If single, isolated ginsenosides are tested, it is impossible to comprehend the adaptogenic effect (page 33) of ginseng. When ginseng adapts its effects to the needs of the organism, the two main groups of panaxdioles and panaxtrioles take on different responsibilities. Whereas panaxdiole Rb1, for example, has a calming effect on the central nervous system, panaxtriole Rg1 has the opposite effect and is therefore stimulating. The different components of the individual ginsenosides of the two main groups are thus held responsible for the various effect profiles. They seem to be the reason why American ginseng has more calming yin energies whereas Korean ginseng is characterized by the more stimulating yang qualities (see also page 31). Therefore, the effect of ginseng cannot be traced to a single isolated ingredient. It can only be explained by looking at the distribution and the interplay and of all the ingredients.

Every group has different duties.

Protection from Age-Related Damage

Biologically active substances were isolated not only from the fresh ginseng root. A phenolic compound, maltol, which is not active in the fresh root, was found in red ginseng (page 25). It is only transformed into a biologically active form during processing. It is believed that maltol protects connective tissue cells from oxygen-related damage and holds back the aging process.

Constituents of the Ginseng Root

Specific Active Agents

Panaxdiole group Ginsenosides	Ra1, Ra2, Ra3, Rb1, Eb2, Rb3, Rc, Rd, Rg3 (+ Rh2, Rs1, Rs2—only in red ginseng)
Panaxtriole group	Re, Rf, Rg1, Rg2, Rh1, Rho
Oleanolic acid	Ro
Phenoles	Maltol (only in red ginseng)

Nonspecific Active Agents

Vitamins	Vitamin B-12, folic acid, nicotine acid, pantothenic acid, biotin, nicotylamide
Mineral salts	Copper, calcium, magnesium, potassium, sodium, phosphorus, iron, aluminum,
Trace elements	Nickel, manganese, chromium, zinc, selenium, molybdenum, cobalt, vanadium, germanium
Amino acids	Aspartic acid, glycine, alanine, proline, valine, isoleucine, tyrosine, phenylalanine, fatty amino acids, arginine
Ethereal oils (0.05 %)	200 separate components
Fats	Neutral fats
Sugar (5%)	Glucose, fructose, saccharose, maltose, trisaccharide

Ginseng—the Joy of Healing

A favorite among young and old

Most Westerners are only familiar with ginseng in the form of capsules that are taken starting at a certain age, often along with vitamins and other tonics. In China and Korea, however, ginseng is not only a remedy for the silver years but also a constant part of daily nutrition. It complements and enriches the diet for adults and children alike. Asians simply enjoy eating and drinking ginseng products, and they find that daily tasks and duties are more easily accomplished with its help. Ginseng is used as a spice and drunk as tea, and whole root pieces are chewed for hours. There are even ginseng cigarettes. Because ginseng is also believed to have moisturizing properties that enhance elasticity, it is used in cosmetics and skin-cleansing products as well.

The Range of Ginseng Products

There are as many different products of ginseng as there are various levels of its quality. The scope of ginseng products that can be obtained in Germany, for example, ranges from fresh roots, extracts, and capsules to teas and schnapps.

Looking Out for Origin and Content

Not all products contain everything that is promised on the label. Everyone who buys ginseng—regardless of the form—should inquire about the origin, the methods of processing, and the active agent content before purchasing it. Cultivation and preservation methods play an important role. High-quality ginseng is obtained in selected regions, like northeastern China and South Korea, by means of traditional cultivation methods (see also page 19). On pages 51 through 55, you can find concrete tips about what you should keep in mind when buying certain products.

There are major differences in active agent content and processing.

Fresh and Dried Ginseng Roots

● *Fresh ginseng* is a rarity in Europe and seldom available. The roots arrive individually packed and vacuum-sealed from their countries of origin, but they are usually used for demonstration and decoration purposes by specialists and pharmacies. These fresh roots are not recommended for consumption. They generally contain large amounts of preservatives and possess no authorization as pharmaceuticals, as opposed to other ginseng products offered in certain countries. You cannot determine the purity and the active agent content simply by looking at the outside of the root.

Vacuum-sealed fresh roots: rare and not always suitable for consumption

● *Dried roots* are usually offered untreated or enriched with bees' honey. Some have notches carved into them in order to make it easier to measure out the required dose. The daily amount is simply broken off at the notch and chewed.

Dried roots have to be chewed for a long time.

■ Dried ginseng roots are usually very hard and difficult to bite into. In order to consume the recommended active agent content, you would have to chew on the root piece for a long time and be sure it mixes well with your saliva before swallowing it. The dried root is therefore not suitable for practical daily use in the West. Dried roots in the

Stuffed Chicken and Honey Roots

In Asia, fresh ginseng is used in many ways. It is prepared as tea or can be added to alcohol. This is how ginseng wine or ginseng liqueur is made. Fresh ginseng also refines food. Ginseng-filled chicken, for example, is popular. Honey ginseng is used as a healthful candy: Whole root pieces—fresh or dried—are marinated in honey for several weeks. Over time, the root soaks up the honey and turns golden-brown and relatively soft. Separate pieces are then chewed and mixed with saliva for a long time. That way, the active agents can be released slowly and absorbed by the body.

Effective
and
practical:
dried roots
in powder
form or as
an extract

form of powder or other drug products, such as capsules, extracts, and extract powder, are easier to consume and medically
more effective.

Powder and Capsules

● *Loose ginseng powder* is a common product, because it is used
in traditional Chinese medicine. To prepare it, dried ginseng
roots are tested for their purity, finely ground, and packaged as
loose powder or filled into capsules. The powder can be consumed pure with some fluid, dissolved in drinks, or sprinkled
over food.

● The most common form of intake, however, is *capsules*. Hard
gelatin capsules that can be opened easily are often used. That
way, you can also consume the active agent in its pure form if
you wish to do so. This is especially helpful for people who find
it difficult to swallow pills or capsules.

Dosages in capsules can be easily measured, because there is
always the same amount of active agents in each of them. The
individual capsules are also vacuum-sealed until consumption. In
comparison to extract or extract powder (see page 43), capsules
dissolve only a little bit later in the stomach and
release the active agents there. This has no
impact on their effectiveness.

■ Capsules are especially useful when
you are travelling. They also have a
neutral taste, so they are suitable
for people who find the typical taste of ginseng too
strong.

High-quality
ginseng
powder in
capsules
can be con-
sumed
easily with
water.

Extract and Extract Powder

Extract and extract powder contain active agents in a concentrated form.

When extract or extract powder is produced, a higher concentration of active agents can be obtained than with normal ginseng powder. Depending on whether they are processed in the cultivation area or somewhere else, the fresh or dried roots are chopped up and placed into special extraction machines. Alcohol or a mixture of water and alcohol is used to aid the extraction of the valuable ingredients from the root. Afterward, the extraction substance completely evaporates. What remains is pure ginseng extract, which is thickened until a red-brown, glutinous extract is obtained, similar to sugar-beet syrup.

It contains all the active ingredients. Traces of pesticide that might be present are removed during the extraction process. If more fluid is evaporated from the extract, a powder is obtained, the so-called extract powder. The typical ginseng taste is preserved in extracts and extract powders. It is slightly bitter, with a sweet aftertaste, and reminds one of the pharmacist's real licorice.

● *Thick extracts* are the preference in naturopathy. The daily dose is consumed pure or brewed up with hot water and drunk as tea.

● The good, highly concentrated *extract powder* and ginseng granules have an especially strong taste. Therefore, it is advisable to prepare them as tea and sweeten them with honey, if desired. But you can also consume the powder in its pure form, letting it dissolve slowly on the tongue. True ginseng fans apparently swear by this! It just comes down to a matter of preference.

Extract powder is often sold in vacuum-sealed portion bags.

■ Extracts and extract powders can be measured out in exact doses and are soluble, and the active agents are absorbed quickly by the mucous membranes. It is important to use up an opened container of thick extract within one to two months. By opening the container again and again to remove the extract, it comes into contact with oxygen or bacteria and can dry out or get contaminated. Extract powder attracts humidity, so it can become lumpy. Therefore, it is also offered in separate, vacuum-sealed portion bags.

Pills and Capsules

● *Tablets* are pressings produced from ginseng granules by mechanical pressure. Tablets contain additional filling, binding, and lubricating substances, and sometimes also colorants. So-called "explosives" help to explode the tablet in the stomach in order to release the active agents.

It's important to look out for the active agent content in ginseng tablets.

● *Capsules* are pressings, like tablets, and are coated with sugar or colored coatings (made out of wax, for example).

■ With tablets and capsules, read the printed matter carefully in order to find out if, or what kind of, additives have been included and how high the active agent content is.

Ginseng Teas

For strength in the midst of daily stress: a cup of ginseng tea

Ginseng tea, sold as instant tea in a powder form, should not be confused with extracts or extract powder, which you can also prepare as a tea. Ginseng tea sometimes only consists of a small part of ginseng extract or granules, and can contain additives, such as fructose or lactose. You can drink it as an accompaniment to your ginseng medication or prepare it to strengthen your defense powers—for example, on cold winter days. You may already like to drink a cup of tea at work, but with a cup of ginseng tea you will treat yourself to something especially good for you in the midst of daily stress.

■ Always store the instant tea dry and well sealed, because it attracts humidity and can easily turn lumpy. Always use a dry spoon when you take it out, and use up the contents of the container rapidly once it has been opened.

Liquid Tonics

Tonic means "strengthening substance."

Tonics are probably the best-known ginseng products. Their active agent content, however, is often only limited, and they contain alcohol. It is therefore necessary to critically assess, in each individual case, if and how they can be used sensibly for medical purposes.

■ Products with alcohol—especially when used continuously—are not suitable for children, patients with liver problems, women during pregnancy or while breast-feeding, and people with alcohol-abuse problems. Always read the label.

Find What's Right for You

It is not possible to say in general which of the many ginseng products that are available will be the right one for you. Every medicinal product has its peculiarities and therefore also advantages and disadvantages in its use. Your choice ultimately depends upon which of the forms of ginseng consumption appeals to you the most and whether you are planning on taking ginseng over a long period of time as treatment or only for a short while.

Cosmetics containing ginseng give one a fresh, clear complexion.

Ginseng in Cosmetics

Ginseng for beauty

More and more cosmetic companies are offering beauty and cleansing products with ginseng. Ginseng helps to increase the moisture level in the skin as well as the elasticity of the connective tissue fibers. Therefore, you can get ginseng in facial creams, lotions, or special cream products, such as eye cream.

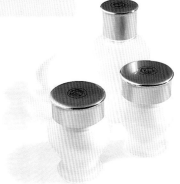

How to Use Ginseng

Measure out the dose according to the active agent content and your personal condition.

As with all herbal remedies, the proper dosage of ginseng depends on the constituents as well as the effect that you want to achieve. Your own condition also plays an important role. You will find more detailed instructions for the different types of application starting on page 61.

Certain fluctuations in constituents cannot be avoided with natural products—and therefore also with ginseng—because every harvest is different. Most producers of extracts, capsules, and tablets, however, pay attention to the relative standardization of the active agent content of their products. You cannot expect such guarantees with fresh roots, though.

Correct Dosage

The German Register of Medicines recommends a daily dose of 1 to 2 grams of dried ginseng root. (One gram is equivalent to approximately one-fourth of a teaspoon.) In order to be able to use the ginseng root in its dried form for medical purposes, the German Register of Medicines stipulates the following minimum active agent content:

Minimum active agent content according to the German Register of Medicines

● At least 1.5 percent of the ginsenoside content, which is 1.5 grams per 100 grams of dried roots. If you consume a daily dose of 1 to 2 grams, this is equivalent to 15 to 30 milligrams of ginsenosides.

● In good roots, the content of ginsenosides can be much higher, though, sometimes between 6 and 8 percent. Even higher concentrations can be achieved through extraction processes: An overall yield of up to 20 percent can be attained with high-quality roots.

This is what the Chinese Register of Medicines suggests.

● The current Chinese Register of Medicines recommends an amount that is three to four and a half times higher: 3 to 9 grams per day, which is equivalent to 45 to 135 milligrams of ginsenosides.

■ Usually, such doses of ginseng do not have any side effects. In Germany, the dosage recommendations of the German Register of Medicines (DAB) are used. The graph below shows you the dosage recommendations of the Chinese Register of Medicines (ChinP) in comparison. When in doubt, consult an experienced doctor or pharmacist.

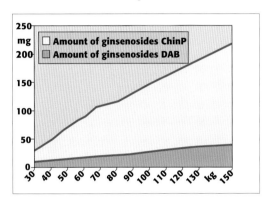

Individual Daily Dosage

Body weight in kg	Amount of ginenocide Average in mgs	
	DAB	ChinP
30	8	24
40	11	24
50	13	38
60	16	60
75	20	72
80	21	90
90	24	96
100	27	108
110	29	120
120	32	132
130	35	144
140	37	156
150	40	168

Calculate Your Individual Daily Dose

Slim people generally respond more quickly to herbal drugs than more corpulent people. Age and our overall health condition also play somewhat of a role. Therefore, you can increase your dose if you are older or heavier. Adjust the generally recommended daily amount of 1 to 2 (or 3 to 9) grams to your needs by converting the given amount to your weight. The numbers in the table are only guidelines, though. You will be the best judge of how much is good for you. Should complications develop, decrease the amount and consult a doctor. (One kilogram equals 2.2 pounds, 1 milligram equals 0.001 grams, and 1 gram is about one-fourth of a teaspoon.)

Always pay attention to you personal well-being.

▶ Special Advice

Make sure that the daily dose of 1 to 2 grams is made from the dried root and that it has

Strength-ening bene-fits through-out the whole day

a concentration of ginsenosides that is as high as possible (see also shopping tips, page 51). You can double the daily dose and consume 2 grams in situations in which you are under a lot of pressure or stress or after an illness or surgery. It is possible to increase the dose even more with products that have a low concentration of ginsenosides. It's preferable to take one-half of the double dose in the morning and the other half at noon. This way, you can make use of the strengthening powers of ginseng throughout the entire day.

Are There Side Effects?

Panax ginseng C. A. Meyer (page 18) is usually highly digestible, even for children (half the dose). If you consume ginseng in regular doses, undesirable side effects or interactions with other medicines are not to be expected. Ginseng has been administered without disadvantageous consequences in Asia for centuries. According to our current knowledge, the long-term use of ginseng medications does not turn into a habit or an addiction. Furthermore, the effect does not diminish over time.

Pay attention to the dosage recommendation.

However, as with other natural remedies, ginseng should not be used carelessly. Even though side effects are usually not to be expected, you are still dealing with a remedy that should be used with care. If too much is taken over a long period of time, even ginseng can have undesirable consequences. Disturbances in the gastrointestinal area are possible because of the high saponin

Inform the Doctor

Speak to your doctor if you want to start a long-term ginseng treatment. This is especially important if you take other medicines regularly or suffer from high blood pressure. Talk to your doctor about the correct dosage, form, and duration of consumption. Doctors of naturopathy or Chinese medicine are particularly well qualified to give such advice.

content. If a great deal of caffeine (such as coffee, tea, or Coke) is consumed at the same time as high doses of ginseng, nervousness can develop. This, however, happens very rarely.

Short- and Long-term Medications

Depending on whether a medicine or a strengthening substance is taken over a short or a longer period of time, one speaks of short-term versus long-term medication.

Short Curative Treatments for Higher Performance and Resistance

More energy and performance strength

If you are young and your body is in good shape, and you find yourself in a situation in which a great deal of mental and physical strength is demanded of you, you can provide yourself with more mental freshness, concentration, and performance strength by starting a short-term ginseng treatment. Examples of such situations are prior to taking an exam, when you have to master an important professional task, and when you are going through quarrels and grief in your personal life.

An Example of a Short Curative Treatment

▶ During special phases of stress, you take the full daily dose (1 to 2 grams, see also page 47) over a period of one to three months. A repeated treatment is possible.

▶ If there is an important task ahead of you, you can start the short-term treatment with a higher ginseng dose (it's best to do this a few days before the actual day). Over a short period of time, the amount taken can be up to two or three times the recommended daily dose, therefore 2 to 3 grams. Decrease the high dose after about three days, and continue with the normal dose.

Strength during stressful situations

Ginseng gives you a boost of energy when you are young. Later on, it strengthens your physical and mental powers.

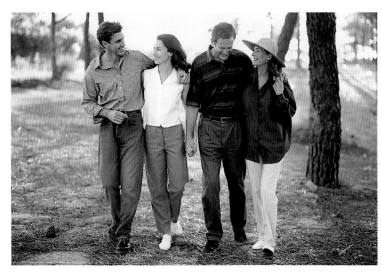

Long-term Treatments—Strengthening Over Time

Even when you are young (say, around 30 years of age), if you find yourself under performance or career pressure, you can take ginseng as a preventive treatment over longer periods. If you are over 40, in poor condition, or suffering from certain ailments (see page 61), it is advisable to take ginseng over a longer period. Ginseng can be used as a long-term medication—for instance, for six to 12 months or even longer.

Prevention in early years

▶ Starting at 30 years of age: When under constant physical or mental pressure, take ginseng daily in reduced amounts—that is, one-third of the daily dose for highly concentrated products (page 51) and the normal dose for those that are less concentrated. Continue this treatment as long as you benefit from it, and repeat it when needed.

▶ Starting at 40 or 50 years of age: A long-term treatment at an older age helps in actively fighting aging. Take the full daily dose of 1 gram with highly concentrated products (about 15 to 30 milligrams of ginsenosides according to the DAB, or 80 to 150 milligrams according to the ChinP, page 47). This should also be the case if you use ginseng as an adjunct to another treatment (for example, in treating diabetes or arteriosclerosis).

Ideal for older people

How to Buy Ginseng

Good advice is invaluable.

In earlier times, ginseng was worth its weight in gold. Today, ginseng is affordable, and it is competent advice that is so valuable, because the variety of products on the market can be so confusing. Good advice can usually be obtained from pharmacies, health food stores, organic food stores, and shops specializing in herbs. Should you be unable to get satisfactory information about specific products from them, turn to the producers themselves if possible. They will gladly send you information about their products' active agent contents, origins, and processing methods.

High-Quality Ginseng Products

Many products to choose from

Ginseng is available in several levels of quality. Fresh and dried roots have active agents of excellent quality, but they are unfortunately not sold in many countries. What's more, it is especially difficult—if not impossible—for the layperson to judge their quality. And not everything that looks like ginseng is truly ginseng.

Products made from red imperial ginseng have a high active agent content.

■ Therefore, you should stick to processed products. The following quality grading is made according to the concentration level of active agents:

● Extract, extract powder, loose powder

● Tablets, capsules, granules, tea

● Mixtures, elixirs, liquid tonics

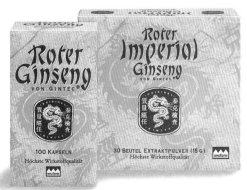

How to Buy Ginseng

Ginseng Type and Origin

When purchasing, be mindful of the place of origin.

● *Panax ginseng C. A. Meyer* (page 18) is recommended for medical use.

● If possible, try to find out where the roots for the specific product come from. Especially high-quality roots originate from the cultivation areas in northeastern China and Korea (see map on page 11). China has considerably larger cultivation areas.

▮ Pay attention to whether it is labeled "red ginseng" or "white ginseng." If you can only find the word "ginseng," it is almost always just white ginseng. Nearly all products in Germany, for instance, are of this root quality.

For the production of red ginseng, only high-quality roots from the best cultivation areas are used, and these roots come from six-year-old plants (see page 25). Red ginseng usually has a high concentration of active agents because of the specific method of conservation. It also contains maltol (page 39).

Active Agent Content and Daily Dosage

● Carefully read the printed matter that comes with the product for the ginsenoside content. The active agent content is ultimately the standard for the quality of a ginseng product. The recommended daily dose lies between 1 and 2 grams of dried roots (remember that a gram is equivalent to about one-fourth of a teaspoon). The active agent content of the products that are offered in Germany, for example, contain between 0.05 and 15 percent ginsenosides.

● When purchasing ginseng, make sure that the active agent content, which corresponds to 1 to 2 grams of the dried root, is included in the particular daily dose (for the active agent content of common ginseng products, see table on page 55). The table on the next page will be helpful in making the conversion.

▮ Always choose a product that contains *100 percent ginseng.* Make sure that no superfluous additives, such as flavors or col-

Conversion Table

Fresh root	Dried root	Root extract
6 grams	1 gram	0.25 to 0.33 gram

Daily dose, according to the German Register of Medicines:

● 1 to 2 grams of the dried root
● 15 to 30 milligrams of ginsenosides at a minimum content of 1.5 percent

Daily dose, according to the Chinese Register of Medicines:

● 3 to 9 grams of the dried root
● 45 to 135 milligrams of ginsenosides at a minimum content of 1.5 percent

Also note the table on page 47.

orants, other remedies, or added vitamins and minerals (ginseng itself already contains a high number of them, page 39) are included. High-quality ginseng is so rich in content and has such a widespread effect that additional substances are not needed. Combinations are sometimes an attempt to compensate for a smaller ginseng content.

■ In Germany, the preferred products have a standardized active agent content and are authorized by pharmaceutical laws, and thus comply with the quality criteria that have been established for medicines there (see page 24).

Drug Products

● Look primarily for extracts, extract powders, and capsules (page 43).

● Tablets often suggest effectiveness, but they actually contain low levels of active agents. They are usually made from cheap root flour, which can be obtained inexpensively on the world market. So, with tablets, pay special attention to the active agent content.

Not only practical at home: Capsules are especially suitable for people who are travelling.

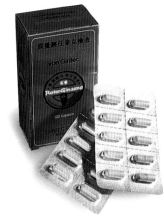

Standardized Active Agent Content

The natural fluctuations of active agent content are balanced through standardization. In order to keep the spectrum of effective substances on a continuously high level, producers have to select ginseng farmers carefully, mix high-quality roots, and guarantee an optimal extraction process. In addition, they must guarantee that only previously analyzed roots will be processed. Independent research institutions ensure the quality of standardized products from the root to the processed product. This elaborate system of quality assurance is naturally costly, but only with such a system can the consumer be certain that the given minimum requirement for active agent content is actually present in every product.

An effective ginseng tea can be prepared from extracts.

● Prepare a tea from tested extracts (page 43). Sachets usually contain minor plant parts, such as leaves. Moreover, the components of sachets do not dissolve immediately in water. It is no wonder that extract producers use elaborate and expensive processes in order to be able to create such genuinely high-quality products.

■ Prices for 1 gram of the dried root can vary a great deal (in Germany, between 1 and 12 DM per gram). The products often drastically differ in their ginsenoside content (0.05 to 15 percent, or 5 to 150 milligrams per daily dose). Therefore, not only is it important to pay attention to the price but also to the relationship between the price and the goods.

High-quality products cost money.

Ginsenoside Content of Various Ginseng Products

The following table will give you an overview of the varying active agent content in common ginseng products offered in pharmacies and health food stores in Germany. A high-pressure liquid chromatography (HPLC) analysis was used to isolate and measure the quantities of the seven most important ginsenosides: Rg1, Re, Rf, Rb1, Rc, Rb2, and Rd.

Ginsenoside Content

Ginseng products (Ginseng producers)	Total ginsenosides in mg (according to 100 g/100ml of the product obtained)
Alsi Ginseng (Alsitan)	4610 mg
Geriatric Pharmaton Vital Capsules (Pharmaton)	120 mg
Ginsana G 115, Fluid (Pharmaton)	38.75 mg
Ginsana G 115, Capsules (Pharmaton)	370 mg
Ginseng "The Active Treatment" (Natura)	383 mg
Grano Vita Ginseng, Strengthened (DE-VAU-GE)	930 mg
Gintec Ginseng Tea (Gintec)	1,140 mg
Korean Ginseng Tea Instant (Hanil)	810 mg
Kumsan Ginseng, Fluid (Much)	63.03 mg
Kumsan Ginseng, Capsules (Much)	1,117 mg
Reform-Ginseng Elixer Plus (Boerner)	1.93 mg
Reform-Ginseng Extra Strong, Fluid (Boerner)	15.82 mg
Reform-Ginseng Capsules "Extra Strong" (Boerner)	1,140 mg
Reform-Ginseng Capsules N (Boerner)	190 mg
Red Ginseng Extract of Gintec (Gintec)	6,470 mg
Red Ginseng Capsules of Gintec (Gintec)	6,310 mg
Red Imperial Ginseng of Gintec (Gintec)	13,940 mg
Sanhelios Ginseng Capsules Plus (Boerner)	170 mg
Tai Ginseng Capsules (Dr. Poehlmann)	340 mg
Tai Ginseng Fluid (Dr. Poehlmann)	57.48 mg

Source: Addipharma GmbH, an analytical research laboratory for
    remedies and the production of pharmaceuticals, Hamburg

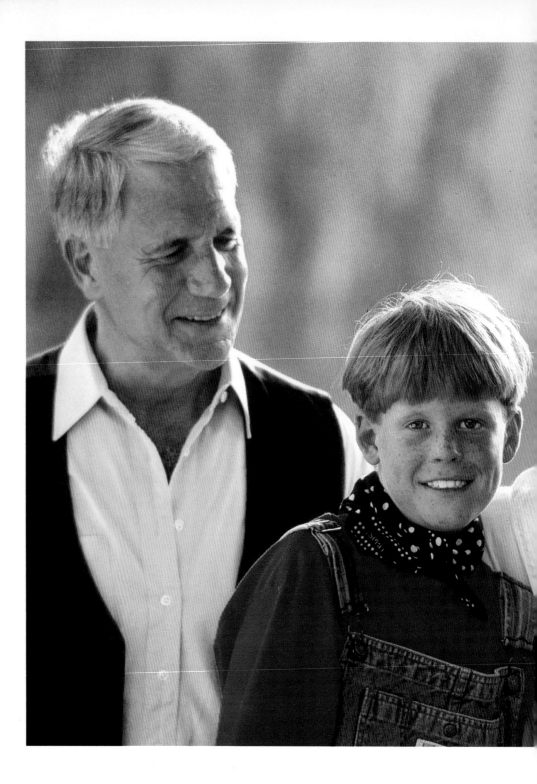

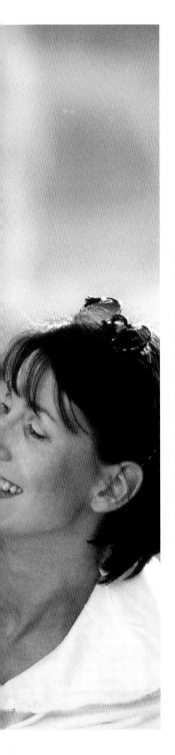

Preventing, Strengthening, and Healing

Ginseng is primarily known as a strengthening substance for older people, because the body needs special support during the breakdown processes. Yet younger people also experience periods of exceptional pressure. Ginseng helps children and teenagers concentrate better at school and in their studies. Adults receive the necessary balance that is needed to master the periods of stress in their private and professional lives. You can strengthen your immune system with ginseng as well as treat a range of specific ailments. Ginseng is also beneficial as an adjunct in the treatment of serious illnesses and accelerates the healing process.

Restoring Balance

Increasing internal and external pressures

Every day many of us have to cope with higher performance demands, strict deadline pressures, and continuous internal tension. In addition, our diets may not be balanced enough, we may exercise too little, and we may be exposed to rising environmental pollution. Children today are increasingly experiencing cardiovascular problems as well as allergies and skin disorders. The high number of psychosomatic illnesses shows how easily body and soul can lose their balance. Many people feel under constant pressure, generally feel unwell, tired, and lacking in energy, have difficulties concentrating, or are barely able to handle their daily tasks.

It is important not to simply accept these problems but to take the alarm signal that your body sends out seriously. Then, in order to eradicate the problem, you need to find out ways that you can bring about changes and improvements in your daily life. Try making use of the far-reaching effects of ginseng. Use it to:

Listen to the body.

● Increase your mental performance

● Deal with stressful situations more easily

● Strengthen the organism against environmental pollution

● Generally get through the day

How Ginseng Helps

You will find out, in the following pages, how ginseng can help you in concrete situations. If not stated otherwise, the ginseng being referred to is the genuine ginseng, originating from Korea and northern China, *Panax ginseng C. A. Mayer* (page 18).

Because ginseng has been used in Asia for many centuries, our knowledge of its effects is wide and reliable. In addition, numerous international scientific tests and studies have shown how ginseng can help to balance various disturbances.

Researched in many studies

Fast Help with Short-term Treatment

Most people react well to ginseng, especially if they take it over a short period of time (for examples of short-term treatment, see page 49). The greater the level of exhaustion or tension, or the higher the need for energy, the easier it is to observe the effects of ginseng treatment.

Relax and absorb new energy.

Should Exhaustion Continue . . .

Exhaustion is not always just a tedious, irksome condition. It is sometimes a signal from the body that there is an illness causing it. If you continuously feel lacking in energy for no apparent reason, it's important to discuss this with your doctor. Taking ginseng could cover up an underlying illness by improving the symptoms. This would help you in the short term but fail to cure the actual illness. And in the meantime, the illness would go untreated.

Long-term Effects

The effects of ginseng are often not immediately obvious in long-term therapy (page 50). If ginseng is not used as an immediate remedy but administered over a longer period of time to improve chronic or age-related illnesses, or during convalescence, it is possible that you won't experience the effects for some time. This does not mean that help isn't on the way. As a result of the nonspecific effects of ginseng, you will catch a cold much less frequently than normally, generally feel more energetic, and be able to deal with pressure much better. To put it simply, you will become tougher. Step by step, your ailments will disappear—for good.

Nonspecific strengthening effects

Who Can Benefit from Ginseng

If you tell someone that you have started taking ginseng, a typical response might be "Already? You're too young for that!" Or, the person might drop a funny remark about your love life. Ginseng is still seen by many as a strengthen-

Restoring Balance

ing substance for older people or as a magical remedy for increasing sexual potency. After all, the sailors who returned to Europe from Asia during the previous centuries brought with them many a tale about the root that bestows eternal life and virility.

Ginseng creates balance and harmony, and is helpful for people at all stages of life.

Ginseng Helps Both Young and Old

Ginseng is an excellent remedy for many of the complaints

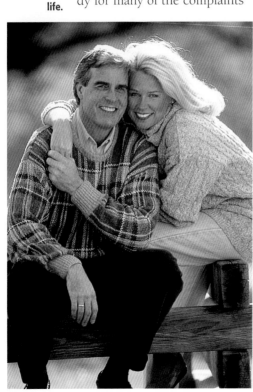

of older people (see page 89). It is also especially important for women during menopause; many of the typical ailments of this period of change can be treated successfully with ginseng.

Teenagers and adults who are in their prime can also benefit from the balancing and healing powers of the royal root.

In the following pages, you will find out about the most important areas of use and learn special tips for different groups of people. The areas of use are categorized in a way that follows the pattern of change that is the basis for the classic Chinese book of remedies *Pen t'sao shen nung* (pages 11 and 29). This pattern consists of:

● *phases of non-change,* your current state with passing disturbances, followed by times of

● *transformation,* which we experience during illness, and, finally,

● *metamorphosis,* such as menopause and old age.

Life means movement and change.

Ginseng for Difficult or Demanding Times

When things get too hard to handle

Everyone can think of times when the daily routine was especially difficult to cope with, when external and internal crises had to be handled, or when one's overall state was critically disturbed. The body rebels against too much pressure—whether from exhaustion, concentration difficulties, headaches, or something else. These disturbances in feelings always serve as an alarm signal. They may not be so severe as to create a serious clinical picture, but they should nonetheless be taken seriously. In Chinese medicine, they are called *phases of non-change*. Ginseng is an important aid during these difficult periods.

Lack of Concentration

Too many impressions and stimuli

Sometimes we simply have to switch off, such as when too much information is coming our way and demanding our attention. Children often have difficulties concentrating as well; they can no longer tolerate all the impressions bombarding them from school, television, computers, and other stimulating sources. But we are not always in the position to create for ourselves the breathing space that we need—be it at school, at work, or in other areas of life.

How Ginseng Helps

Although ginseng doesn't create free time for us, it does release the energy that we

It is important for children to be able work peacefully and stay concentrated

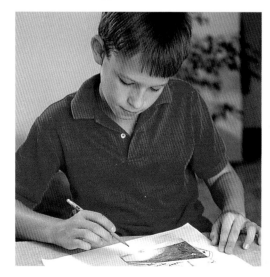

Ginseng Tips

● **For children:** If your children have problems concentrating or are taking many exams, give them half a daily dose of ginseng (half a gram)—for example, extract powder or a bit of extract with honey—for one week. You can serve them tea prepared with the extract powder and sweetened with honey before they leave for school.

● **Below age 40:** A short-term ginseng treatment is appropriate during particularly stressful periods (page 49). You can start with a higher dose (2 grams of the dried root). After one week, continue with the normal dose of 1 gram as long as it is helpful.

● **Age 50 and above:** Take ginseng daily for several months at the same dose of 1 to 1.5 grams (the equivalent of 30 to 150 milligrams of ginsenosides).

Taking up and storing stimuli

need for thinking. Our alertness increases, and our ability to comprehend is stimulated.

Ginseng influences mental performance in many positive ways. It is not completely clear how this works, although ginsenosides Rg1, Rg2, and Rb1 (see page 37) are held responsible. They measurably increase the reaction time of nerve cells, so that stimuli can be more quickly digested and passed on.

Quicker Reactions

In 1956, the ginseng researcher Petkov discovered in experiments that trial candidates who had taken ginseng had quicker reactions to certain cues and could give correct answers more rapidly than those in a neutral control group. They were also quicker at learning new vocabulary words and could use them more effectively. Other tests with radio operators showed that they, too, had faster reactions with ginseng.

Quicker and better reactions

What Else You Can Do

Although ginseng helps you perform better mentally, it is important in terms of holistic medicine to approach everything from several angles, so give your brain some time to rest when it needs it. Lack of concentration can be a completely normal reaction to external pressures or psychological problems.

● Sometimes planning the day better already helps in putting the mind at ease. Try making up a list of all your daily duties and then thinking about which ones you can eliminate.

● Perhaps a certain issue is worrying you so much that everything else recedes into the background. If you find that you can't handle the problem on your own, don't hesitate to make use of therapeutic help.

● A well-trained memory can still work well in old age. The blueprint: Be mentally active, talk to others, learn new things, and perhaps participate in a mental-training program with other people.

The brain also rests during sleep. A short nap of about 20 minutes around noon can be especially refreshing.

Stress

Everyone is familiar with the sensation: You feel numb, yet energy is pounding underneath at the same time, and the mouth gets dry, the blood pressure goes up, and the pulse is racing—stress hormones are being released. That is how the human

Stress can block thinking.

organism often reacts to threats and danger. This is the case when the trigger is a psychological crisis or an external pressure—a wild bear doesn't have to suddenly appear before us. Other than in nature—where, for instance, antelope mobilize their resources to escape the tiger—the alarmed condition of the whole organism is given little credence in our modern civilization. The adrenal cortex hormones that are suddenly released in great quantities are not discharged properly by a reaction of the body, meaning by flight or attack. The human organism is well prepared for short-term stress, which can even inspire us. However, our bodies react to constant stress frequently with exhaustion and insomnia, because the constant mobilization of all our resources is exhausting and draining even if we are not being challenged physically.

When pressure turns inside

How Ginseng Helps

Ginseng has a twofold effect on stress:

● In an acute situation, ginseng increases one's physical

Ginseng for Difficult or Demanding Times

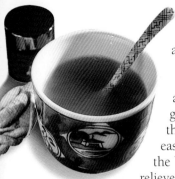

and mental performance.

Ginseng helps to activate the energy transmitters in the blood more easily. This is how the body gets relieved, because the existing energy can be used better.

In times of stress, ginseng extract can also be prepared as tea.

● Once the stress has passed, ginseng helps to reduce the physical stress symptoms more quickly. Ginseng reduces the production of the alarm substances in the adrenal cortex. In addition, the glucocorticoids in the system are broken down more efficiently in the liver. The metabolism returns to its normal pace.

Mobilizing and Relaxing

Various tests have shown that ginseng can mobilize existing energies while having balancing and calming effects at the same time. It has been reported that Chinese and Vietnamese soldiers carried pieces of ginseng root with them during the Indochina war so that they would not collapse from stress and shock after being wounded.

Dealing better with pressure

Ginseng Tips

● **Short periods of stress:** You should consume double the daily dose in predictably stressful situations (2 to 4 grams): 1 to 2 grams in the morning, 1 to 2 grams at noon, both before meals. Afterward, continue taking the normal daily dose of 1 gram for another couple of weeks.

➤People who are extremely stressed or travel a great deal are advised to take capsules for practical reasons.

● **Continuous stress:** During long phases of stress, you can take ginseng over a longer period of time. But it's also important to remember to find some moments of relaxation during times of prolonged stress. Prepare ginseng extract or powder as tea, and take a few minutes to drink it in peace. Enjoy this short ritual.

➤Instead of drinking cups of coffee in stressful periods, replace the coffee with ginseng tea from time to time (page 44).

What Else You Can Do

Realize the limits of your ability to cope with stress.

Anyone who suffers from continuous professional or personal stress places demands on his or her body to accept more than it can handle, usually with harmful consequences. Ginseng can help the body to deal with stress more easily. But even with ginseng, there are limits to a person's ability to cope.

● This is why you should try to relax as often as possible. Auto-suggestive training is an excellent means of building up energy in the meantime. Health centers and adult education programs offer courses.

● Physical exercise is a great way to reduce stress. Try to find an exercise program that you can easily incorporate into your daily schedule. This can be a short aerobics class or half an hour of swimming in the closest swimming pool. Often an evening walk in the fresh air (at least 30 minutes) can be enough.

Exercise daily—it balances things.

● Look at whether you are trying to escape stress with too much alcohol and nicotine. Remember that men

should not consume more than 40 grams of pure alcohol per day, which is about two bottles of beer or two glasses of wine (0.4 liter). Women can cope with less. For them, the limit is 30 grams of pure alcohol. These days there are a lot of ways to quit smoking. The best method is often to do this with others in a course (your doctor or a health center should be able to recommend one).

● You can learn to plan your day better. If you find this difficult to do by yourself, there are courses and books that offer valuable advice.

Walking is an especially effective way to reduce stress and improve one's overall condition.

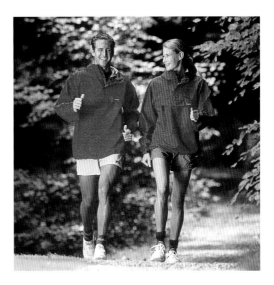

Exhaustion and Fatigue

If life energy (yang) is at a low ebb

There may be days when you just don't feel up to it. Perhaps you don't even want to get out of bed or you want to stay at the breakfast table forever. General exhaustion is a sign that you are consciously or subconsciously asking more from yourself than you are able to give at the present time. A doctor of Chinese medicine would probably diagnose you as having a lack of yang, or life energy (page 30).

How Ginseng Helps

Regain your strength— for good.

Ginseng can help you use your strength carefully and economically. Ginsenosides have a gently strengthening effect, unlike stimulants that give you a false sense of energy. With ginseng, you will rediscover your lost strength. Ginseng is calming but at the same time doesn't reduce your driving power. You will feel fresher. Ginsenosides and their various adaptogenic effect mechanisms work together:

Investigate Possible Causes

Fluctuations in a woman's monthly menstrual cycle, the remains of the flu, or simply advanced exhaustion can be reasons for chronic fatigue. But chronic fatigue could also be a signal of an illness, so if you have felt weak for a long time you should discuss this with your doctor.

● The availability of the body's own energy carriers is increased. The sugar level in the blood rises by a small amount.

● At the same time, only the energy that you actually need is released by normalizing the heart function, circulation, and metabolism. Your internal system works more economically.

Quicker Recovery

Animal tests and clinical studies have shown again and again that periods of convalescence after extreme exhaustion are much shorter with ginseng. Another effect, increasing physical performance, has been shown by clinical tests with athletes, seniors, and nurses.

In one study, night nurses received 1.2 grams of root powder at the beginning of their shift. It was clear that the nurses didn't become as tired as they usually did and felt fresher than normal when their night shift was over. They also completed their tasks with more energy, reacted better, made better-aimed decisions, and created a more positive working atmosphere.

A better mood at work

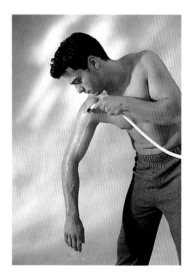

Ginseng Tips

In comparison to other substances, such as caffeine, ginseng is not a stimulant. It strengthens and supports the body and has balancing qualities.

● **For immediate effects:** When needed, take a double dose—that is, 2 grams—for a short time (three days). Afterward, cut back to the normal daily dose.

● **For older people:** Many older people have successfully gotten over their fatigue and lack of energy by taking ginseng regularly over several years or in regular intervals. Chronic fatigue, however, should always be discussed with a doctor!

What Else You Can Do

● Supplement your newly gained energy by taking regular walks or jogging in the fresh air.

● Targeted breathing exercises will also give you energy. Alternating from hot to cold water during your morning shower, as well as dry brushing, will get the circulation going.

➤ *Another tip:* Ethereal oils can be used to combat fatigue. Mix a few drops of rosemary, ginger, juniper, and peppermint oil in a cup with sweet cream for a refreshing bath oil.

A stream of cold water running across the arms quickly eliminates fatigue: Start at your wrist on the outside, bring the stream up to your shoulder, and then run the water back to the wrist but on the inside of your arm.

Better Performance

There are challenges in our lives that we want to face well prepared. An important job interview, a decisive competi-tion, or a strenuous mountain hike make us think of ways that we can multiply our physical and mental resources.

How Ginseng Helps

The performance-improving effect of ginseng is traced to various ginsenosides, espe-cially the components of Rg1, Rg2, and Rb1 (see page 37). The muscles receive more oxygen while the body is in action. Waste products, such as lactic acid, that are generated during muscle exercise and normally lead to stiffness are broken down more quickly.

Running Faster

During a test in the fifties, a hundred young soldiers had to race against each other. Half of them had consumed a ginseng product a few hours earlier; the other half had ingested a placebo product that tasted similar (a product without active agents). The group that had the ginseng finished noticeably earlier than the group that had not received the treatment.

Ginseng improves perfor-mance.

Ginseng Tips

● **Short term:** Start taking a double dose (2 grams) two or three days before the important deadline. Distribute intakes evenly between morning and lunch. Then, depending on your condition, continue taking the normal dose for a while longer.

● **Long term:** If you have to perform well over a longer period of time, you should take ginseng at the normal dose (1 gram per day) for several months. *If you are under 40,* after an initial phase of one to three months you can reduce the normal dose by half (1/2 to 1 gram) and then continue taking it for a longer period of time for sup-port and prevention. *If you are over 40* or once the overall level of your performance starts to decline, you can take 1 gram per day (page 91). A product with a high active agent content is best. Although this will not make you immortal, it will give you back your vigor.

Impotence

Sexual problems are more frequent than is commonly thought. Women often complain about a lack of desire, whereas many men experience problems with erection already at a young age. If lovemaking doesn't work out as one wanted it to a couple of times, these experiences can affect one's self-esteem and sense of well-being and lead to internal tension and fear of failure. Male sexual disorders can have both physical and psychological causes. Apart from disturbances in hormonal balance and deficiencies in metabolism (diabetes), strained nerves and stress are the main causes of temporary and chronic impotence.

More often than not, temporary sexual problems turn into a vicious circle: Afraid of another display of impotence, a man succumbs to internal pressure, and this additional stress then impedes his erection the next time he makes love, or leads to an early ejaculation.

How Ginseng Helps

Forget about the idea that ginseng will increase your sexual performance; don't think of it like a magic substance or use it with any sense of shame. Ginseng is not a sex drug. But if you try to find a solution by restoring your inner balance, it can often be of help. This is true for:

● People who are under a lot of pressure in their daily lives and/or relationships. With ginseng, they are helped to perform more effectively and stay more relaxed. Ginseng also releases energy, and this too has a positive effect on one's sex life.

**Leave the
tension
behind, and
rediscover
the excite-
ment of
love.**

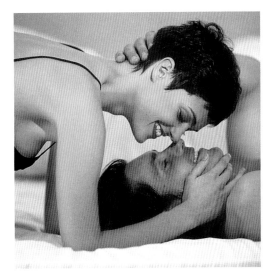

● People who have a disturbed hormone balance. They benefit from the regulating adaptogenic effect of ginsenosides (page 37).

● People with metabolic problems. They profit from an improvement in metabolic functions.

It regulates and balances.

● Older people, who will benefit from the regulating and strengthening effects of ginseng. The release of life energy, yang, also includes sexual energy and increases sexual desire.

A Resurgence of Sexuality

Japanese doctors have discovered that a man's sperm count increases after the consumption of ginsenosides; this is similar to the effect of male sex hormones (testosterone). A blossoming of sexual energy has also been detected in older people who have consumed ginseng. Even a renewal of menstruation has been observed in some women.

What Else You Can Do

● It is very important to value yourself foremost as a human being and not as a "performance machine." Make use of other ways to show affection and desire. Only if you stop pressuring yourself will you be able to enjoy making love again.

Try not to put yourself under pressure.

● Openly discuss your problems and desires with your partner. Many problems that hold us back can be resolved in this way.

● Have yourself tested for possible biological causes of your potency problems. An experienced sex therapist can usually help with chronic problems.

● Just like continuous professional or personal stress (page 63), too much alcohol and nicotine can also decrease potency.

Seek therapeutic help.

Ginseng Tip

Support your life energy and therefore also your sexuality by taking ginseng over a period of several months. You will regain your inner balance more easily and feel full of strength and desire again—unless a serious illness is causing your problems.

Harmful Environmental Influences

The environment is very polluted.

Everyone today depends on the external environment in many ways and is exposed in varying degrees to its harmful influences. Environmental poisons come from factories, heavily used roads, and sometimes even our jobs. We may have jobs that are taking their toll on our health, but we can't quit them for financial reasons In fact, many environmental poisons cannot be avoided, so you should try to be prepared for them and deal with them as well as possible.

How Ginseng Helps

Ginseng can help you to lessen the force with which you are hit with pollution and environmental poisons. Many studies have shown that the organism can deal better with harmful chemicals when aided by ginseng.

● This is because ginsenosides strengthen the immune system in general.

● At the same time, they activate enzymes that control the metabolism. This is how harmful substances are eliminated more rapidly, compensating for the damage. The supportive effect is particularly observed in the organs that produce blood.

● The cells are supported in the same way: The time that injured liver cells and blood cells need to regenerate is markedly shorter. This effect applies to all toxins, including alcohol and other intoxicating substances, medicines, and environmental poisons. Even the effects of radioactive pollution can be alleviated by ginseng.

Toxins Are Resisted More Easily

Russian and Chinese astronauts took ginsenosides during their stay in space to protect themselves against harmful influences. Animal tests have shown that ginseng improves one's resistance to toxins and other harmful substances. Because similar tests are fortunately not performed on humans, animal tests are used as an example. However, it was only in those instances where red ginseng was

More strength in combating harmful substances

Ginseng in space

Ginseng Tips

● **Increased strain over a short period:** If you are aware of a situation in which you will be exposed to harmful substances, such as a pending X ray, take three times the normal ginseng dose (3 grams) two or three days before. Stick to the higher dose for an additional day. Afterward, return to the normal amount, and take it over a couple of weeks, so that the body can eliminate the toxins more rapidly.

● **Long-term damage:** Those who live or work in an environment where they are often exposed to toxins should take ginseng regularly, being mindful of the dosage recommendation.

● **Damage from an addiction:** The abuse of alcohol, nicotine, medicines, and other drugs harms the body and the psyche of the affected individual. Often only external help makes it possible to escape the destructive addiction. During and following a detoxifying treatment, such as alcohol detoxification, or quitting smoking, you should plan a ginseng curative treatment so that the toxins that are still in the body will be absorbed more rapidly and the damaged organs will be able to regenerate. Be especially careful in these situations that the ginseng product that is used does not contain alcohol.

administered orally that such effects were demonstrated.

The survival rate of mice exposed to X rays, alcohol poisoning, and otherwise deadly viruses was significantly longer after a ginseng treatment. A weaker effect of cancer-causing substances was also shown. This was only true for substances that did not cause sarcoma (malignant tumors).

Toxins can be absorbed better.

What Else You Can Do

● Your lifestyle can often contribute to your undergoing less damage from exposure to harmful substances—be it by following a diet that is rich in vitamins and miner salts, exercising regularly, or doing relaxation techniques.

You are not completely helpless when exposed to harmful situations.

● Also, find out at work or in your community how you can get actively involved in the protection of the environment.

Illness—a Time of Transformation

Apart from normal situations in life, there are also times when the body has to struggle especially hard to keeps its balance. Illnesses are such times and constitute decisive turning points. In fact, sometimes illnesses may change the direction of our lives.

Illnesses have to be overcome, and the strain, which has developed as a result of the organism's battle with the illness, has to be absorbed.

How Ginseng Helps

Balance and support with ginseng

● Ginseng isn't able to play a major role in the struggle for health in these times, but it is suitable for working behind the scenes, helping patients to collect and concentrate their strengths.

● Ginseng can directly influence the diseases that disrupt the normal metabolism of the body.

Not a Cure-all

Please remember that the regulating effect of ginseng cannot cure the disease that caused the imbalance. Always consult your doctor, and do not use ginseng as a secret wonder drug! Because ginseng strengthens you and diminishes the apparent symptoms, its effect can actually make the diagnosis more difficult.

● A patient's condition can improve significantly through the complementary effect that ginseng has on many diseases, such as cancer, that require intense and often long medical treatment.

The treatment of serious diseases always has to be supervised by a doctor.

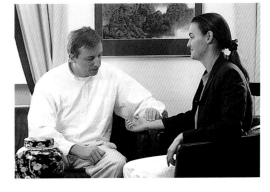

Immune Deficiency

The immune system is under a great deal of strain.

Our bodies not only have to defend themselves against an infinite number of disease-causing agents but also against many different environmental influences. Often it is the coughing passenger on the bus who gets our immune systems going; at the same time, exhaust fumes penetrate the doors, and when we get off the bus, a cold wind blows all sorts of dirt into our noses. In the summer, we can't go into the open air without worrying from time to time about the high ozone levels. Extreme stress and psychological problems also weaken our immune systems.

Stress — Psyche

Chronic infections — Environmental pollution

Medicines — Diet

Intoxicants, drugs — Sleep

Blood circulation

Digestion

Many factors influence the immune system.

Possible Signs of a Weakened Immune System

- You catch colds often.
- You get bladder infections easily.
- You tend to get fungal infections.
- You often get herpes.
- You suffer from allergies.
- You have skin problems.
- You are constantly tired, exhausted, or lacking in energy.
- You recover slowly.

How Ginseng Helps

Ginseng strengthens and mobilizes the body's own immune powers like no other remedy—and, in correct doses—without side effects.

Many tests have shown that, when the body's own powers have been generally improved by ginseng, they can defend us better from physical substances, particles or rays, chemical substances, such as exhaust fumes and tetrachloride carbons, and biological substances, like bacteria and viruses.

Ginseng as an immune curative treatment

Ginseng activates a certain kind of white blood cell, the b-lymphocytes. These produce specific protein molecules, or antibodies, that eventually lead to the destruction of bacteria. Interferon, which hinders the multiplication of viruses, is also produced to a larger extent. Additionally, special defense factors increase in the blood serum.

Certain cells that are active in the liver as well as other defense cells are stimulated so that they increase their desire for food—that is, they increasingly absorb substances that do not belong to the body.

Ginseng Tip

Consider scheduling your ginseng treatment for the wet and cold autumn period. This way, you can reward your body with an internal holiday and give a boost to the energy that tends to decrease around this time of year. At the same time, you will be strengthening your immune system and supporting it in its fight against colds, which we catch more frequently during this period of climactic change. Also, taking ginseng in the fall might save you from a runny nose next winter.

Catching Fewer Colds

In 1972, tests with ginsenosides were conducted with a thousand workers in Siberia. The workers who had taken ginseng caught colds 30 percent less often than those in the control group.

What Else You Can Do

● Take a look at the picture on the opposite page once again. You will probably recognize certain areas with which you especially have problems. Think about which ones you can influence the easiest.

● Think about your diet habits, for example. Or, reflect on which medicines that you take might be unnecessary. It's always a good time to quit smoking (ask your doctor about classes and clinics).

● Try to spend as much time as possible outside.

Headaches and Migraines

Headaches without an apparent cause Those people who wake up with a pounding headache from time to time, feeling as if their skull is going to explode any second, usually know the reason: a heavy drinking session, too little sleep, or simply a change in the weather. However, there isn't always an easily determined cause for this tormenting symptom, and many people regularly suffer from bad headaches or migraines. Painkillers, which are often used, can give some temporary relief, but they **Be cautious when using painkillers.** don't eliminate the causes and might bring about an addiction as a result of frequent use.

There are as many theories about the causes of headaches as there are possible causes themselves. However, there is reason to believe that an insufficient supply of blood in the brain, which could be due to various factors, might be the culprit.

How Ginseng Helps

Ginseng can help profoundly. Ginseng is not a painkiller. In any event, pain is simply an expression of other disturbances in the organism.

Investigate the Causes

It is important to consult a doctor, particularly if the headaches appear frequently and without any apparent reason.

● Headaches are often a signal of another illness (symptomatic headache).

● In addition, there is another kind of headache that cannot be linked to other problems (idiopathic headache).

Ginseng normalizes circulation and reduces the increased tension that causes a tightening of the blood vessels. As a result, headaches are alleviated and appear less frequently. Especially if you have a tendency to get headaches that are not caused by another disease, you can often achieve a lasting improvement if you take ginseng regularly.

Fewer Headaches

Traditional Chinese medicine has successfully used ginseng for a long time as a remedy for headaches, weak nerves, and insomnia. Medical tests have additionally shown that headaches caused by other problems (cardiovascular, for example) were significantly reduced by ginseng.

Headaches often accompany other ailments.

Ginseng Tips

● **Frequent headaches:** If you get frequent headaches and haven't received a clear diagnosis from a doctor, make yourself a cup of tea from ginseng extract and drink it in the morning and in the evening. Make sure that you consume at least 20 to 30 milligrams of ginsenosides per day (following the recommendations of the German Register of Medicines or its traditional Chinese counterpart, pages 46–47), which is a little more than the daily dose of 1 gram of the dried root. Continue this treatment for at least one to three months.

● **Symptomatic headaches:** If your headaches appear while you have another illness, you can usually support a medical therapy with ginseng. Continue to take ginseng for a while after you have finished your therapy. Follow the recommendations above.

What Else You Can Do

● Remember that headaches and migraines are often caused by psychological problems. Think about what bothers you the most, and get therapeutic help, if appropriate.

● Too much alcohol and nicotine, an irregular diet, or too little exercise can lead to headaches. Headache problems will often improve rapidly once you start to make changes in your daily habits.

● Also think about visiting an eye specialist. If there is too much strain on your eyes or you suffer from a problem with your sight, headaches often develop as a result.

● Consider your posture and working habits. You can reduce tension with specific exercises and by balancing your movements.

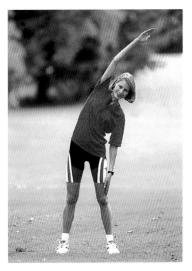

Regular exercise in the fresh air helps reduce tension.

Diabetes

Handling the illness

Fortunately, people suffering from diabetes can lead relatively normal lives these days if they receive insulin regularly and stick to a special diet. *Diabetes mellitus* includes all the illnesses that are caused by an increased blood-sugar level or by an insufficiency in metabolizing carbohydrates in a reasonable time frame. A deficiency in insulin, a hormone of the pancreas, is the cause of it. Symptoms of diabetes are increased thirst and a decrease in the capacity to perform both physically and mentally.

How Ginseng Works

Ginseng can support the body's own insulin production in the insular cells of the pancreas and improve carbohydrate metabolism at the same time.

Ginseng supports diabetes treatment.

Ginseng is used to support the treatment of diabetes, because it naturally improves the effect of therapeutically administered insulin. On a practical level, this means that the external addition of insulin can usually be reduced. Ginseng also lessens certain symptoms of diabetes, such as ringing in the ears, cold fingertips, and the common feeling of exhaustion.

The effect that is similar to that of insulin does not stem from the ginsenosides so much as from a short protein molecule and a carbon acid contained in the root. However, these active agents have been isolated only recently, so they have not been examined very closely yet.

Reducing symptoms

Less Insulin

The Japanese scientists Okuda and Yoshide observed 21 diabetes patients over a period of three months. The overall clinical picture of 12 patients improved after they received ginseng-root powder. Three patients did not need insulin any longer, and five others managed with a reduced dose. The other four patients experienced an improvement in their blood pressure, in the eye damage caused by diabetes, and in the shoulder pain caused by the illness.

Ginseng Tip

Diabetics in particular suffer from fatigue and lack of energy. They often feel better generally with ginseng, which normally fosters more energy. It is advised to take ginseng as an adjunct to your long-term therapy—after talking to your doctor—in a dose of 1 gram per day.

What Else You Can Do

● A diet that includes a great deal of fresh fruit and vegetables is especially important for diabetics. Enjoy eating healthily and within limits. Mediterranean cuisine, which contains lots of vegetables and plant oils, is especially suitable for diabetics. Reduce meat, eat more fish instead, and replace sweets with fruit. Above all, put love and time into your cooking!

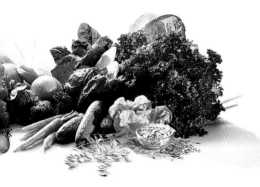

● Diabetics should be active and exercise regularly. This is how the blood-sugar level is reduced.

Cancer

Every person has cancer cells, but they do not necessarily cause cancer. Only once the balance of the immune system is disturbed can they actually multiply and cause the typical clinical picture that we know as cancer. Physical as well as psychological factors play an important role in the development of cancer. In acute cases, the immune system is partly responsible for whether tumor cells can cause tumors (metastases) in other places or not.

Physical and psychological factors play a role.

Cancer significantly reduces energy levels, especially during the late phase when lethargy and a numbing exhaustion are pervasive.

How Ginseng Helps

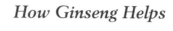

Like mistletoe, ginseng cannot cure tumors, but it can still be of additional help. Ginseng stimulates the immune system due to its many active agents.

Ginseng supports the immune system.

● For a healthy person, ginseng reduces the possibility of getting cancer, because cancerous cells are combated by an effective immune defense.

● During the early stages, a stronger immune system not only prevents the development of tumors but also of cancer. This is how you give your body a break so that it can regain its energy.

A break to get back energy

● Someone with cancer will have a bit more time to relax and breathe because of the gently energizing effect of ginseng.

Influencing Tumor Growth

The success of ginseng in preventing the growth of tumors partly stems from the increase in the powers of the immune system. Today, the possible use of a glucose-protein molecule (high-polymeric peptidoglycan) recently discovered in the ginseng root is being considered; however, its effect is not yet fully known.

In addition, ginseng constituents have been shown to slow down the growth of certain tumor cells. This is partially due to the fact that ginseno-

sides, and Rb2 in particular, log on to steroid hormone receptors that are effective in the cells. A slower cell division has been observed in cultures. Tests with animals have shown a higher survival rate after ginsenosides have been administered.

Coping Better with Therapy

More often than not, the necessary cancer therapy, with its strong medications (chemotherapy) and radiation treatment, places additional strains on the patient's already weakened organism and immune system. Ginseng helps the body to adjust more easily to the serious tumor therapy. It supports the detoxification process of the liver and helps the damaged liver cells in regenerating more quickly. Blood production is stimulated, and white blood cells are supported in their battle against the damaging influences (see also page 83).

Tests in Japan have shown that patients who received ginseng in conjunction with chemotherapy were doing much better. They felt better in general, had fewer prob-

Giving the organism additional strength

lems, regained their appetite more quickly, and gained weight faster. In addition, hemoglobin, responsible for the transportation of oxygen, increased, as did lymphocytes and immunoglobulins, which are important for resistance.

Better blood results

Preventing Cancer

The cancer-preventing effect was studied with 905 test couples in 1990. There were 13 percent fewer cases of cancer in the group that had been taking ginseng than in the control group. It was also shown that extracts and the root powder provided better

Ginseng Tips

There is still no cure for cancer. Prevention, however, is especially important with this disease.

● In addition to other preventive measures, regular curative treatments with ginseng extracts (pages 43 and 50) can support your body and possibly prevent tumor cells from growing.

● If you are in treatment, it's advised to take high doses of ginseng extract over the entire duration as well as during post-treatment care—after discussing this with your doctor.

protection than fresh roots.

What Else You Can Do

● Trace elements, such as manganese, iron, copper, zinc, and selenium, strengthen your immune system and are already contained in high-quality ginseng roots in their natural form (pages 36 and 39). A diet mainly consisting of organic food, which is also rich in trace elements, helps in prevention as well. It's also important to eat lots of fresh fruit and vegetables.

An adequate and balanced diet

● Even when you take ginseng, it is essential to have regular checkups for cancer. If cancer is recognized early, it is easier to treat and the chances of recovery are considerably higher. The most important checkups are testicle examinations for young men between the ages of 20 and 35 and prostate, skin, and large-intestine examinations for men over 45. Women should get their genital organs checked when they are 20 years of age, their breasts and skin when they are 30, and their large intestine when they are 45.

The importance of regular preventive checkups

Recovery

The body and the psyche together have to cope with the consequences of an illness.

Illnesses not only impair our well-being for a certain amount of time, but they also frequently are decisive events and bring about changes in our lives. Recovery is the transitional period between an acute illness and normal life.

After the body has been weakened by an illness, it has to regain its strength and deal with the aftermath of the illness. During such times, you are not actually sick anymore, but you are also not very well equipped to handle stress. It takes some time for the body and the psyche to overcome the consequences of an illness or an injury.

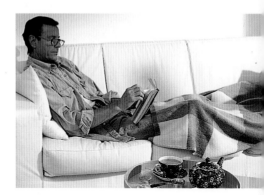

● Perhaps you had to take medication during your illness that helped your body defeat the disease. However, many medications have undesirable side effects, and they have to be dealt with along with the illness itself. Ginseng helps the organism eliminate harmful substances or waste products that have been produced.

The organism needs time to regain its strength.

How Ginseng Helps

Faster recovery with ginseng

● Ginseng is especially helpful during the period of recovery, whether from an infection, surgery, or an injury. Ginseng improves the functioning of the metabolism, so that your body has more energy to heal itself. At the same time, ginseng supports the immune system, which has been weakened during the illness or injury.

More Energy for Body and Psyche

Ginsenosides, especially Rb1, support the metabolism of nerves and muscle cells, and therefore improve their performance level. Ginseng strengthens the heart and circulation, and the heart rate is increased. At the same time, ginsenosides stimulate the body's own defense system in general. Therefore, pathogens and harmful waste products can be eliminated from the system more quickly and can be broken down more efficiently by the kidneys and the liver. Furthermore, the uplifting, energizing effect of ginseng helps in raising your overall mood as you recover more rapidly.

The psyche is also strengthened.

Better Blood Levels

A study of 120 patients who had taken ginseng after gynecological surgery showed that the number of leukocytes (white blood cells) and the overall serum protein had improved significantly. In addition, the women who took ginseng gained weight more quickly than those who did not.

Patients who received therapeutic radiation of the bone marrow also recovered much better when taking ginseng, as blood platelets were produced in higher numbers.

Better recovery in patients

What Else You Can Do

● During recovery, make sure to follow a diet that is easily digestible and rich in vitamins and minerals.

● Gradually resume your physical activities. Ask your physician what kind of exercise is best for you. If possible, do not return to a hectic daily schedule right after an illness. An illness can be seen as a sign that something is changing and starting anew in your life. The period of recovery is also a time of reflection. If you experience the period of recovery consciously, this could be an opportunity to organize your life in a more satisfying way.

Make use of the recovery period.

Ginseng Tips

● Take time to recover from your illness. Make use of ginseng to regain your energy, and support your body with a long-term ginseng curative treatment (page 50). Pay special attention to high-quality products, such as extracts or extract powder (page 43).

● Consult your physician after a serious illness or surgery. Do not follow the prescriptions of traditional Chinese medicine during a fever or acute infections, but only once they have started to recede.

Arteriosclerosis

Arteries can already harden at a young age. Most of the time, however, fat from the blood only starts to build up on the walls of blood vessels when we are older, hardening the artery walls. High cholesterol levels make this more likely to happen. Blood can flow through a healthy artery without any problems. A hardened artery demands higher heart activity, because the necessary blood amounts can only be circulated by increasing pressure (high blood pressure) and a higher beat frequency (pulse).

Frequently arteriosclerosis is accompanied by a deficient blood supply to the heart and the brain. The risk of a heart attack or a stroke is therefore doubled. Thromboses can also develop, because blood gets lumpy.

Increased risk of heart attack or stroke

How Ginseng Helps

Ginseng is generally a suitable remedy for preventing arteriosclerosis. It stimulates enzyme activities that participate in the metabolism of fats so that less residue is made in the vessels. Ginseng consumption aids the transformation and absorption of cholesterol.

However, ginseng cannot eliminate or cure the damages that have already been inflicted upon the arteries. But it reduces strains that you are exposed to and postpones and reduces sclerosis.

Prevention through ginseng

● Ginsenosides optimize the energy level—the way this happens under stress (page 63). This is how the pulse rate can be reduced.

● Rg1 lowers blood pressure

What You Should Know About Cholesterol

Cholesterol is basically important for the organism. It supports cell growth and enables the production of gall acids, hormones, and vitamin D. Cholesterol can be produced by the body (in the liver), but is mainly gained through food. Animal fat, egg yolks, and entrails are especially rich in cholesterol. But your cholesterol level should remain within certain limits. Protein components play an important role in that respect. Too much "bad" transport protein LDL supports fat deposits, whereas HDL keeps blood fats at a healthy level. Consuming too much fat can, among other things, lead to a high cholesterol level in the blood.

Participating in a sport that you enjoy is another way to counter-act deposits in the vessels.

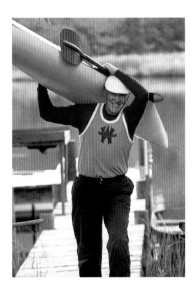

reduced in your vessels. Because the HDL level (see box, page 84) remains unchanged or increases, ginseng is helpful in maintaining an overall balanced cholesterol level.

Reduce existing damages.

and helps in loosening blood vessels—as far as this is possible considering the deposits that are already there.

● Ginseng improves the metabolism. This means, among other things, that nutrients are absorbed and transformed into energy whereas harmful substances are eliminated more quickly. This is how the heart and the brain can be supplied with oxygen better and longer.

● With ginsenosides Rb1, Rb2, Rg1, and Re, the more damaging kind of cholesterol (LDL) is absorbed by the liver and taken out of blood circulation. This way, deposits are

Ginseng Tips

The danger of arteriosclerosis should be taken seriously. It would be a mistake to think that a spoonful of ginseng will allow you to continue to "sin"—that is, to persist in smoking, eating too much fat or eating too heavily, and not exercising regularly. Use ginseng, such as high-quality extracts, in regular treatments to help your body deal with the "old baggage." What's more, a change in your diet that is recommended by a doctor will be much easier to handle with the energizing effect of ginseng.

What Else You Can Do

Remember, you are as old as your blood vessels. They can already harden at a young age. However, you can take small steps that will help you lead a healthy but no less enjoyable lifestyle.

Less meat and more vegetables

● Discover the joy of cooking, and try out vegetarian dishes more frequently. Many restaurants offer alternatives to pork roast, such as salad bars.

● Buy low-fat products—there are tasty variations, especially for milk products.

● And finally, take the stairs instead of the elevator once in a while. This will also help your arteries.

Cardiovascular Disorders

Keep your heart and circulation going.

The heart and circulation keep our bodies going. They are the engines of life. Because of our way of life these days in modern cities, we do not keep the heart and circulation in shape by exercising them in the various ways we would in a natural environment. Cardiovascular diseases are therefore some of the most common diseases in modern civilization, as well as some of the most common causes of death.

Signs of High Blood Pressure

High blood pressure becomes apparent through serious headaches, difficulties in breathing during stress, nosebleeds, ringing in the ears, and mental confusion. Heart asthma, sight problems, and angina pectoris can develop later. Blood pressure is high once it exceeds 160 mm Hg (systolic pressure) and goes below 95 mm Hg (diastolic pressure).

High Blood Pressure and Its Consequences

Our hearts beat 10,000 times per day and pump out between 5,000 and 7,000 liters of blood. Blood pressure is the power that develops when the heart muscle is contracted in order to keep blood circulation going. Blood constantly has to overcome a certain resistance in the blood vessels. The smaller the vessels, the more pressure has to be exerted by the heart for the metabolism to function. Increased blood pressure is the result. But certain organic disorders, such as a kidney disorder, can cause high blood pressure as well. The heart and blood vessels can be damaged because of the constant strain, just like those organs that are receiving less

Damages from poor blood circulation

blood. A heart attack, kidney failure, a stroke, and, in the worst-case scenario, a brain hemorrhage are some of the possible and dangerous consequences.

How Ginseng Helps

Ginseng does not save you from regular trips to the doctor and from blood-pressure checkups, but it can strengthen your heart and its performance.

● The metabolism of the heart muscle is improved, so it can function more easily. Unlike other remedies that support the heart muscles, the pumping performance is not increased for a short time but rather improved in the long run.

Ginseng Tips

Never treat your blood pressure on your own. But you can support your organism with ginseng. Remember that the effect can be reversed: Once you stop taking ginseng, your blood pressure can increase again. Therefore, a long-term treatment with a high-quality ginseng extract is advisable (pages 43 and 50).

● Ginsenosides, especially Rb1, cause a relaxation of the blood vessels and thus lower blood pressure.

What Else You Can Do

● If you have high blood pressure, it is especially important to follow a low-sodium and low-fat diet and to watch your weight in order to lessen the strain on your organism.

**Make it
easier for
your heart
to work.**

● Sports, such as cross-country skiing, jogging, walking, biking, and swimming, are advantageous for people with high blood pressure.

Other Illnesses

There are numerous other illnesses for which ginseng has proven to be especially effective. Its use in the practice of traditional Chinese medicine as well as experiences with its use in Western countries have shown this. But there's nothing like first-hand experience to see if regular ginseng consumption will help you with certain problems or in particular situations. Ginseng was shown to help in the follow-

**Ginseng can
help in the
healing
process of
many ill-
nesses.**

Become more resistant.

ing areas. However, consult your physician regarding serious illnesses.

● **Allergies, neurodermatitis, acne**
Ginseng stabilizes the body's own protective mechanism, and it can reduce itches and rashes.

Energized and more active with ginseng

● **Gout and rheumatism**
Ginseng regulates uric acid metabolism. Complaints can be reduced.

● **Depression**
Ginseng boosts energy levels in general, lessens insomnia, and activates those energy levels that are responsible for motivation and drive, thereby counteracting depression.

● **Gastrointestinal problems**
Intestinal movement and digestion are improved. Ginseng makes the distribution of fats easier, whereas the absorption of sugar is slowed down. This is especially important for diabetics (page 78).

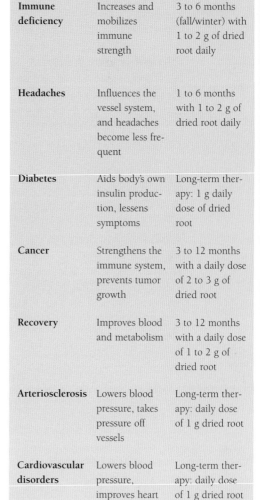

Ginseng Treatments in a Nutshell

Ailment	Effects	Treatment
Immune deficiency	Increases and mobilizes immune strength	3 to 6 months (fall/winter) with 1 to 2 g of dried root daily
Headaches	Influences the vessel system, and headaches become less frequent	1 to 6 months with 1 to 2 g of dried root daily
Diabetes	Aids body's own insulin production, lessens symptoms	Long-term therapy: 1 g daily dose of dried root
Cancer	Strengthens the immune system, prevents tumor growth	3 to 12 months with a daily dose of 2 to 3 g of dried root
Recovery	Improves blood and metabolism	3 to 12 months with a daily dose of 1 to 2 g of dried root
Arteriosclerosis	Lowers blood pressure, takes pressure off vessels	Long-term therapy: daily dose of 1 g dried root
Cardiovascular disorders	Lowers blood pressure, improves heart performance	Long-term therapy: daily dose of 1 g dried root

Maturity—a Time of Metamorphosis

Accepting the cycle of life

Life is an ongoing cycle in which we move on and mature. If we can open up to the ideas of maturation and metamorphosis and accept them with equanimity, we will experience happiness and harmony and stay young in our hearts. Ginseng is often helpful in this respect.

Menopause

Body and psyche have to readjust.

Menopause is not only a period of physical changes for women. Women undergo hormonal changes that put an end to their biological ability to procreate, and this causes fluctuations in their physical and psychological states that can be strong or weak.

Women sometimes suffer from hot flashes, get dizzy, and feel less energetic. More fat is deposited around the stomach and the hips. On the psychological level, some women experience insomnia, irritation, and depression. These typical ramifications are caused by the difficulties that the hormone system encounters in its attempts to readjust itself. The hormone production, which regulates processes in the ovaries, fallopian tubes, and the uterus, is slowly shutting down. The hormone balance is off. Every woman faces these changes. But this does not necessarily mean that all women have to endure the discomforts that frequently accompany them.

Those who consciously and positively prepare for a new stage in life discover new possibilities and strengths.

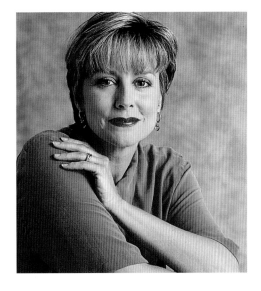

How Ginseng Helps

If you take ginseng during menopause, you will soon feel more energetic physically and more balanced emotionally. In addition, ginseng helps the hormonal system to adjust more easily to the new condition of the body. The adjustment happens more quietly and in "softer" waves.

Easier adjustments

● Ginsenoside Rb1 can improve muscle and tissue metabolism, so that energy can flow more easily again. Because of this, you will feel more relaxed and generally fresher, more energetic, and less irritable. You will also cope with mood changes more easily.

● The release of hormones from the pituitary gland and the adrenal cortex is controlled in a beneficial way. Hormones FSH and LH, which are produced there and are responsible for the interplay of the sexual hormones (estrogen and progesterone), can adjust to their absence more quickly.

● These fluctuations in the hormonal system can manifest in hot flashes. Ginseng decreases the number and strength of such reactions.

Fewer hot flashes

Feeling Better

Studies have shown that women who consumed a high-quality ginseng product during menopause suffered significantly less from typical occurrences, such as nervousness, hot flashes, nocturnal sweats, and headaches. They were generally in a better mood, slept better, and had fewer problems with their sexuality.

Ginseng Tips

● **Long-term treatment:** It's advised to take ginseng all through menopause, either regularly or in regular intervals. It supports the body and the psyche. Even if a long-term treatment with a high-quality product (page 50) might seem expensive, it is worth it because it will protect your nerves and generally make you feel more energetic. Take 1 gram of ginseng extract or extract powder every day before breakfast.

● If you are traveling, take 2 or 3 capsules daily. Make sure that you receive the daily dose of 1 gram of dried ginseng.

➤ **Extra tip:** Drink a light ginseng tea instead of alcohol at night in order to sleep better. You should avoid alcohol in general during menopause.

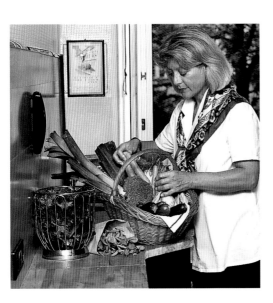

Old Age

People are getting older and older but not necessarily in a healthier manner. Many elderly people complain that they are tired, feel weak, and lack energy. In addition, they often suffer from various ailments. With old age, the organism starts to be less reliable: The blood pressure changes, the metabolism is unbalanced and decreases, the number of cells in the central nervous system lowers, and the hormones are not as finely tuned as they once were. People are prone to get sick more easily in old age. The performance level is down, and many things that did not pose problems before become strenuous and taxing. Therefore, older people should be conscious of using the energy that they do have sparingly and of making the best use of it.

Healthy cooking is fun, and fresh vegetables provide you with important vitamins and minerals.

What Else You Can Do

It is important to get enough calcium during menopause in order to prevent osteoporosis. Change your diet, if necessary. For example, replace:
● meat with cheese during breakfast and dinner,
● meat with vegetables that you cover with cheese for lunch, and
● cake with yogurt.
    It's also a good idea to drink mineral water, which is rich in calcium (500 mg Ca/l). By doing this, your calcium level will rise dramatically.

Elderly people need to use their energy economically.

How Ginseng Helps

Ginseng is a remedy that is especially well suited for old age. It is generally refreshing, supports the important physical functions, and increases performance levels.
    The organism can work more economically by using the energy it still possesses in a

Ginseng activates and supports.

way in which it actually conserves it. Because ginseng relieves the heart and blood circulation and improves the oxygen supply, mental performance is improved as well. You may not feel young in your old age, but you can certainly retain some youthful vigor.

Saving energy

● Ginseng ensures that the blood vessels remain permeable and elastic (see page 85), and also slightly lowers the number of heart beats, so that the heart is relieved of pressure.

● The hormonal activity of the adrenal cortex is stimulated as is therefore that of the metabolism. The increased energy also brings about a greater joy in living along with a heightened sense of mental well-being.

Feeling and reacting better

● Ginsenoside Rg1 ensures that the central nervous system processes impulses in a better way. This is important for your ability to concentrate and react in old age.

● The aging of cells is slowed down particularly by the presence of maltol in red ginseng (pages 25 and 38). Produced during the Maillard reaction in the preservation process, maltol protects the body from oxygen-related cell damage.

● Once the whole organism is relieved in its functioning, not only will you be able to perform better but you will also experience positive mood changes.

More Joy in Living

Studies in nursing homes have shown that their residents—with an average age of 72—who took 0.7 grams of the

Ginseng Tips

The body readily accepts support from ginseng during old age, because ginseng stimulates gently.

● **Ginseng taken over a long period of time:** It is preferable to take highly concentrated ginseng as an extract or extract powder (page 43) on a regular basis. If you are concerned about the expense, lower the dose rather than give up the long-term consumption and its curative effects. Of course, it's important to discuss your ailments with your doctor.

● **No additives:** Make sure that the products that you will be using over a long period of time contain ginsenosides in effective amounts (see also pages 46 and 55) and do not have any additives that might dilute the purity of the product. Trials have shown that ginseng works better when consumed in its pure form.

root powder for a period of more than 100 days were significantly better in their performance than a group that had received a placebo. The members of the ginseng group were able to remember more and displayed a better imagination. They felt a greater joy in living, and their ability to express themselves was much higher. In addition, age-related ailments, such as insomnia, dizziness, a pounding heart, and nervousness, decreased.

Calmer and more focused

What Else You Can Do

Exercise is especially important in old age. You do not have to expect records from yourself. Especially enjoy activities in nature. And they can even be more enjoyable with others. The following activities are particularly suited to older people:

A reasonable amount of exercise and a balanced diet are good for your overall well-being.

- Low-impact aerobics
- Swimming
- Hiking
- Walking
- Tennis
- Dancing

Many ailments that affect older people can be prevented with a balanced diet that includes a lot of fresh vegetables, a sufficient amount of whole-wheat products, and mainly vegetable fats (like sun-

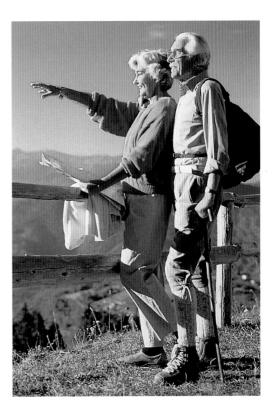

flower and thistle oil), but little salt, alcohol, and coffee. It is also advisable to eat less in general: The caloric needs of women between the ages of 25 and 65 decrease by about 20 percent, from 2,200 to 1,700 calories; those of men between the same ages decrease by about 25 percent, from 2,600 to 1,900 calories. Naturally, the amount of calories you should consume depends on your height and weight and also on how physically active you are.

Hiking and enjoying nature together promotes a sense of joy in living.

About This Book

About the Author

Ernst D. Prinzenberg, born in 1939, is a pharmacist and studied pharmacology in Würzburg, Germany. His interests include natural chemistry in connection with folk medicine. He has worked for many years with the ginseng root and gathered scientific material and reports on actual experiences.

Photo and Other Credits

Bavaria: 50, 61, 93; Berwanger: 31; BlasÈ Agentur: 56/57; Faltermaier: 65, 77; Gintec: 8/9, 10, 12, 14, 15, 16, 20, 19, 21, 33, 35, 37, 51; Jahreis: 73; Kollnflockenwerke: 79; Masoni: 69, 74; v. Salomon: 67; Studio Schmitz: 26/27, 29, 41, 42, 43, 44, 45, 53, 64, 82, 88, 91; Stock Market: 32, 60, 85; Tony Stone: 89

Graphics: sXe-Grafik
Map: Kartographie Huber

Index